ESSIAC

The Secrets of Rene Caisse's Herbal Pharmacy

By the same authors

Essiac Essentials: Rene Caisse's Herbal Cancer Remedy (1999)

Essiac

The Secrets of Rene Caisse's Herbal Pharmacy

Sheila Snow & Mali Klein

Newleaf

Newleaf
an imprint of
Gill & Macmillan Ltd
Hume Avenue
Park West
Dublin 12
with associated companies throughout the world
www.gillmacmillan.ie

© 2001 Sheila Snow & Mali Klein

0 7171 3228 5

Index compiled by Kate Duffy
Print origination by
Carrigboy Typesetting Services, Co. Cork
Printed by ColourBooks Ltd, Dublin

*The paper used in this book is made from the wood pulp of managed
forests. For every tree felled, at least one tree is planted, thereby
renewing natural resources.*

A catalogue record is available for this book from the British Library.

1 3 5 4 2

Contents

*'If it has no value, why are they so concerned
if I take it to my grave?'*
Rene Caisse, 1978

Introduction

*I*f Essiac had been expensive to produce, Rene Caisse would never have been able to afford to give it away. If Essiac had been difficult to make, she would never have been able to manufacture the decoction in the quantities necessary to treat the hundreds of people who came to the Bracebridge Cancer Clinic during the 1930s. If Essiac had shown no merit the clinic would never have existed and the Canadian government would never have wasted time and money investigating her work.

Those of us who have become involved in researching Rene Caisse's Essiac are all aware that we have not been achieving results on the same scale as she did. From the evidence of the government records alone there can be no doubt that Essiac works. We know there must have been something more in addition to the basic four-herb recipe, the 'something more' that achieved the sometimes spectacular results recorded at the Cancer Commission Hearings of February and July 1939.

Making full use of Sheila's unique access to archive information as a result of her association with Rene during the last years of her life, combined with Mali's active, hands-on experience with Clouds Trust, UK, we returned to the lake in Canada at midsummer exactly two years after writing *Essiac Essentials* to find that elusive 'something more'.

Essiac Essentials encourages self-sufficiency, detailing the basic, step-by-step recipe preparation, how to make Essiac, what to look out for and how to identify, locate, grow and harvest the four herbs to make up the tea. *Essiac – The Secrets of Rene Caisse's Herbal Pharmacy* expands the vision to develop the research and to reveal what we have discovered of other formulae and herbs Rene used or may have used alongside the basic four. This includes previously unpublished material concerning Rene's Kidney Pill formula and the Sheep sorrel solution she used either topically, as an enema, douche, mouthwash and by injection, alongside the basic four-herb decoction during the Bracebridge clinic years. The archive has also revealed hitherto unknown information concerning the roles played by some of the more prominent figures involved with Rene and Essiac, particularly during the last years of her life. In addition, we have included information on the basic science of cancer, the related chemical and radiation therapies and the importance of maintaining a healthy diet and lifestyle to enhance the general understanding of the possibly palliative and remedial effects of the Essiac formula.

Once again as the authors, we must state that the book has been written simply to present the facts according to the results of our combined research. We have no intention of making any claims concerning the remedy, and we do not endorse any particular commercial product.

A well-respected Essiac researcher recently wrote to say 'there is a kind of magic between Sheila Snow and Mali Klein'. We have endeavoured to bring that magic once more into what we intend to be our ultimate book about Essiac. This time we are truly handing on the torch.

Chapter One

Essiac – The Basic Recipe

*R*ene Caisse's basic Essiac recipe uses four commonly known herbs – powdered Sheep sorrel (whole herb), chopped Burdock root, powdered Slippery elm inner bark and powdered Turkey rhubarb root – to be prepared as a decoction and taken diluted in water and sipped as a tea. Rene had reversed her family name to describe the simple herbal formula she had developed from the original eight-herb recipe given to an Englishwoman with breast cancer by an unknown Native American herbalist in northern Ontario at the end of the nineteenth century. The reports recorded at the two Canadian Cancer Commission Hearings in 1939 describe results that might be considered almost miraculous by today's standards, when cancer patients were treated primarily with a combination of the basic Essiac decoction as an oral therapy and a Sheep sorrel solution given by injection. Rene spent the rest of her life until her death aged ninety in 1978 trying to make Essiac readily available 'to people, not just to research animals', as she often said.

Since the recipe was published, many people living with cancer are using Essiac or an Essiac derivative, very often with their doctor's approval, as so many admit their patients appear to do well when taking the remedy and show no signs of harmful side effects. However, there are a bewildering number of Essiac derivative products currently available commercially, and many claims have been made. Our combined research has convinced us that Rene's basic formula is still the best, and then only when careful attention is paid both to the quality of the herbs and the quantities used in the recipe. People who are ill have a right to the best of whatever it takes to give them every chance to get well, and anyone who chooses to take Essiac has a right to the best herbs prepared exactly as Rene prepared them in the 1930s. As she said, 'If it works, don't change it.' Essiac worked for Rene Caisse; it can work for us now.

So who had the recipe?

We cannot begin to write another book about Essiac without first establishing who may have inherited the correct information from Rene Caisse before she died, while demonstrating our sources of credibility and reference. We know Rene wrote down the original eight-herb recipe when she met the elderly English lady in 1922. Rene went on to develop the basic four-herb Essiac formula during the 1920s with the help of a team of doctors in Toronto. Recognition must be given to one, Dr Robert Fisher, who was particularly interested in what she was doing and made several key suggestions to facilitate her research.

There is no evidence to prove that Rene ever wrote down the Essiac recipe again until the period covering the last 18 months of her life after the first major article about her work was published in the Canadian *Homemakers Magazine* in June 1977. Given the extreme secrecy of her nature and the fear of prosecution for apparently practising medicine unlicensed that dogged her for most of her working life with Essiac, it is highly unlikely that she would have ever trusted the knowledge anywhere outside her own head. Charles McGaughey, her husband of five years, left no indication that he knew the formula, and his surviving family have never revealed any knowledge of the recipe.

We believe that Rene wrote down directions for Essiac for the first time when she prepared the sealed version of the recipe to present to Lieutenant-Governor Pauline McGibbon on 15 August 1977, to hold in trust until 'the results of treatment of cancer patients at two Canadian cancer clinics are known'. Rene told a journalist from the *Toronto Star* that she 'decided to give up her remedy after reading articles in the media which depicted her as an old lady unwilling to share the remedy to help humanity'. The unopened envelope containing the Essiac formula was returned to Rene in October, hours before she sold a version of the formula to the Resperin Corporation from Toronto for one dollar.

Archive information lists the possibility of five individuals and two commercial companies who were linked with Rene Caisse during the vital, final two years of her life, any one of whom may have genuinely gained access to the Essiac formula.

MARY McPHERSON
Mary knew Rene over a period of 43 years. Initially she helped collect signatures for the series of four petitions requesting that Rene be granted special permission to continue to develop her work with Essiac. These petitions were presented to the Ontario parliament in Toronto annually over the period from 1935 to 1938. In the later years, Mary helped with making up the Essiac when Rene was no longer physically able.

Although Mary and Sheila were both visiting Rene regularly during 1974 to 1977, they never met at her house and did not become friends until 1988 when Sheila visited Mary, needing Essiac for a friend. Towards the end of that year, Mary handed Sheila a long white envelope with 'To my dear Mary' written in pencil in Rene's handwriting on the front.

'I don't want this any more. You can have it,' said Mary.

Sheila opened the envelope and took out an old and tattered piece of paper folded into three. It was a photocopy of the rough copy of the handwritten version of the Essiac formula Rene was preparing for the Resperin Corporation before the contract was signed in the autumn of 1977. Mary had made the corrections to the recipe as Rene was writing it out. We have reproduced the paper exactly as written, including Mary's amendments and corrections.

'Sorrel no longer used as hypo injection but put in the Oral medication as a complete Oral treatment for Cancer.

5lbs powdered Burdock root – "coarsely ground and 5 8oz. cups" added in Mary's writing.

1 ounce India rhubarb – "turkish" written over India, "Turkish is better" in brackets, both added in Mary's writing.

1lb powdered sorrel.

1 quarter pound slippery elm bark.

Red clover blossom 1 quarter pound – words scratched out, "added, not in Essiac" in Mary's writing.

Watercress 1 quarter pound.

Perrywinkle 1 quarter pound – words scratched out, "added, not in Essiac" in Mary's writing.

All ingredients powdered and mixed.

1 ounce of the mixed ingredients to be put into 32 ounces boiling water for ten minutes.

Remove from heat and cover.

Let stand for eight hours or overnight then drain, do not strain into bottles and seal.'

When Mary pointed out the differences in comparison to the recipe she was used to making up for Rene, particularly concerning the Burdock proportion, Rene laughed and said, 'Well, they'll have to come and ask me about it, won't they?'

By 1977, Rene had carefully guarded the secret of the recipe for 55 years. She always said 'once you write something down, you've lost it'. Finally she found it very difficult to let Essiac go. She had never trusted anyone else to give the formula the same meticulous attention to detail either in preparation or administration, and she was anxious to remain part of the research team as long as she could. Unfortunately, once she had signed the agreement, 'they' never came to talk to her about the recipe again.

Resperin's Dr Matthew Dymond asked Mary to teach him to make up the recipe after Rene's death. Mary later signed an affidavit in Bracebridge in December 1994, entrusting the document to the Bracebridge Town vault. Copies are on view in the library and in the Rene Caisse room in the basement of the Woodchester Museum in Bracebridge. Mary is a unique witness to Rene's life and work. We have no reason to doubt her version of the recipe as given.

DR CHESTER STOCK (VICE-PRESIDENT FOR ACADEMIC AFFAIRS, MEMORIAL SLOAN-KETTERING CANCER CENTER, NY (MSKCC))

Rene sent samples of the Sheep sorrel herb, excluding the three remaining herbs, to Dr Stock for research. She kept up correspondence with him from 1973 to 1976, at last using the opportunity to write freely and confidentially since she felt that he was the 'one person I could trust to prove my long years of work'. She used the series of letters to outline the recipe for the Sheep sorrel solution for injection and sent supplies of the herb together with samples of the solution prepared in ampoules, which could have been at least 14 or 15 years old at the time of use. However, she found correspondence by letter limiting and frustrating, especially as Dr Stock steadfastly refused either to meet her or to talk with her over the phone. She was never invited to visit the research laboratory.

Sheila was invited to visit Dr Stock personally at MSKCC on 11 February 1977 while she was compiling information for the *Homemakers* article, due to be published the following June. Two years later, after Rene's death, Sheila contacted Dr Stock once more, asking for copies of Rene's letters for archive information. Accordingly he sent her photocopies of most of the letters, using his discretion in withholding those written in stronger language which clearly revealed Rene's annoyance at how the research was being conducted. Having carefully examined the evidence from the letters, we have no reason to believe that Rene ever gave Dr Stock the full Essiac recipe. She was still refusing to send the three remaining herbs to him as late as 1977.

CORMAC PUBLICATIONS – HOMEMAKERS MAGAZINE

Sheila had been taking notes and compiling material from Rene's written archive information since they were introduced to each other by the local doctor in September 1974, intending to publish an article that might initiate a book about Rene Caisse and Essiac. Both *Chatelaine* magazine and *Reader's Digest* rejected Sheila's first attempt at writing the article in the autumn of 1976. Early in January 1977, Jeffrey W. Shearer, executive vice-president of *Homemakers Magazine*, contacted Sheila to suggest that she might collaborate on a full article with Carroll Allen, the head of the food department at *Homemakers*. Sheila would provide the direct link to Rene and verify the research.

Carroll and Sheila interviewed Rene regularly during the first three months of 1977. On 3 March, Sheila witnessed an interview between Rene and Jane Hughes, the editor of the magazine. Carroll Allen and a lawyer representing Cormac Publications, the company responsible for *Homemakers Magazine*, were also present. Jane had been instructed to ask Rene to consider signing a contract with *Homemakers* to set up a trust fund to promote and research Essiac. The trust would apply for a patent on Essiac and bid for facilities to research the formula. Essiac would remain under Rene's control and supervision during her lifetime, all rights reverting to the trust after her death. Rene became anxious when Jane admitted that the contract depended on her finally revealing the formula and asked for more time to think about it. True to character, she called the magazine several days later to say the deal was off.

Neither Sheila nor Rene had seen the finished article when the magazine sent out pre-publication copies without their knowledge to a list of doctors for comment and feedback. Not one of the doctors had a good word to say in Rene's favour, one commenting that he considered the magazine to be instrumental in perpetuating a fraud. Already feeling badly let down and betrayed, Rene was very offended when she read the descriptions of 'her vivid flowered dress' and her 'masses of costume jewelry' and 'herbs sat cheek by jowl with daiquiri mix' in the fridge. She burst into tears and said to Carroll, 'I want you to tell Jane Hughes that this is the most malicious story I have ever read about me.'

Rene was initially outraged and resentful when the magazine article was published and later flattered by the sheer volume of attention she received. There is no evidence to prove that Rene ever gave the recipe to anyone involved with Cormac Publications.

RESPERIN CORPORATION

David Fingard, head of Resperin Corporation, first contacted Rene on 13 August 1977 when an increasing number of people were trying to persuade her to reveal the ingredients of the recipe. Rene never liked David Fingard. She found him arrogant, disorganised and rudely dismissive of the doctors who were working with him. Sheila was accidentally witness to the meeting between Rene and the Resperin representatives on Monday, 5 September 1977 at Rene's house in Hiram Street, Bracebridge. David Fingard, accompanied by his wife, Mildred, and three doctors – Wilson, Rynard and Dymond – called to discuss the possibilities of drawing up a contract with Rene to give Resperin the exclusive rights to market Essiac. Rene's lack of respect for David Fingard did not extend to the doctors; she was impressed by their seeming sincerity in offering to set up six research clinics across Canada.

The contract was signed on 26 October 1977. Confident of being invited to take part in setting up the research and marketing programme, Rene was saddened and disappointed as she found herself increasingly isolated and no longer able to take an active part in the work. In a taped interview a year later, in June 1978, when she was asked how she felt since the secret of the Essiac formula was no longer her own, she replied 'I feel lost without it.'

The confusing evidence of Rene's handwritten recipe given to Mary in October 1977, together with Mary's own oral and written evidence, suggests that the original Resperin version of the Essiac formula may have contained a larger proportion of Burdock than Rene customarily used when making up the formula herself. In the early years Resperin produced the decoction in glass medicine bottles. When they changed to plastic packaging during the 1980s, several people reported to Mary saying the tea tasted awful and they were nervous about using it. David Fingard died in 1989.

We visited Mary in the local hospital in Bracebridge on 5 July 2000. She was as bright and 'feisty' as ever and told us about an evening meeting two weeks previously to which she had been invited to as a guest of honour by the company that was continuing the Resperin Corporation work with Essiac.

'They had the Town Crier and the whole bit,' she told us. 'I sat there, checking out what they had to say about Rene, making sure they got it right. I didn't want them to think she was some backwoods grandmother who cooked up a stew.'

We began to laugh and she added, 'And when that fella was talking to me about the Essiac, I told him "you got the right ingredients but you don't make it like she did". It went past him like a breeze, like it always does.'

GILBERT BLONDIN

Sheila walked into Rene's house on a Saturday afternoon in August 1977 to find Gilbert Blondin decorating the kitchen. He was one of the few people Rene found she could rely on at that time. He drove down to Bracebridge every week from Hull, Quebec, about 300 miles each way, to collect Essiac for his young wife who was desperately ill with acute leukaemia. Sometimes his brother drove with him to help renovate and repair Rene's house. Occasionally one of his friends came too.

Rene liked having Gilbert around because he gave her time and he met his commitments. When he said he was going to visit, he came promptly and did exactly what she expected him to do. He started making up his own Essiac shortly after Rene died. Sheila tasted his version of the formula in 1985, when he went into partnership with Dr Pierre Gaulin, and she remembers it as having the correct 'tang' of the Sheep sorrel. The colour of the tea was good and the price reasonable at that time.

It must be remembered that Rene was never one to put all her eggs in one basket. In 1977 she was 89 years old, she was nervous about the Resperin contract and she didn't trust David Fingard. Gilbert Blondin's wife had made a remarkable recovery and Rene trusted him. We have no reason not to believe that Rene gave him the recipe before she died.

PAT JUDSON

Gary Glum was having dinner in André's Restaurant in Bracebridge with Mary and her husband in the fall of 1988, after completing a book signing for *Calling of an Angel* in

Scott's of Muskoka bookstore. Mary and Cliff McPherson and several other people were witnesses that evening to Gary Glum's statement that he had bought a version of the Essiac recipe from Mrs Pat Judson of Deering, Michigan who was currently president of the Foundation for Alternative Cancer Therapy (FACT) chapter in Detroit.

We know that Pat visited Rene in late 1977 wanting Essiac for herself and one other person. She returned once again the following March 1978 accompanied by her husband and Resperin's David Fingard. By then she was involved in a class ation suit in Detroit, demanding the right to have access to Essiac in that city. Pat came to Bracebridge with her husband in August 1978 for Rene's 90th birthday celebrations, and we believe Rene could have given Pat a version of the recipe either then or later in September 1978 after Rene had travelled to Detroit to receive an award at the FACT convention. Mary later verified the version of the recipe Pat had given to Gary Glum. We have no evidence to doubt his claim.

DR CHARLES BRUSCH

Dr Brusch was undoubtedly a well-intentioned man, but we believe his part in the Essiac story has been grossly exaggerated. Rene briefly joined forces with Dr Brusch to research Essiac at the Brusch Medical Center in Cambridge, Massachusetts in May 1959. Their active collaboration ceased in June 1960 when the supply of research material and resources to the Center was suspended. There is no record of any further correspondence between Rene and Dr Brusch until his letter of 21 September 1976, headed 'Brusch Medical Center', apologising for not having contacted her for so long as to be completely out of touch with her and her work with Essiac.

Dr Brusch and his wife Jane maintained correspondence with Mary and Sheila after Rene's death, exchanging a total of 29 letters over the period from 22 February 1979 to the last letter from Jane to Sheila dated 14 July 1994, almost nine months after Dr Brusch's death in October 1993. We have used extracts from these letters to back up our hypothesis that Rene

Caisse never divulged the Essiac formula to Dr Brusch. This is compounded by Mary's report of having witnessed the telephone conversation between Rene and Dr Brusch in October 1977, just before the contract with Resperin Corporation was due to be signed when Rene offered to give him the formula and he refused her offer. A few days later Dr Brusch flew in to Toronto to act as an independent witness to the contract when it was signed.

In 1979, Dr Brusch received a letter from the Massachusetts Medical Society dated 13 March summoning him to appear before the Committee on Ethics and Discipline on 8 April to answer a complaint against him 'concerning the use of certain herbs in the treatment of cancer'. He was asked to provide: 'complete evidence of the Essiac formula used in your herb tea. This should include evidence that you have indicated in your letter of the Canadian government's determination on the safety and efficacy of this material.'

On 22 March Dr Brusch sent a letter to Sheila with a request for

'any copies of information you (Sheila) have of research done in 1974 by Sloan-Kettering Company, especially reports that reveal testing results, proving that Essiac is non-toxic, that patients using Essiac had regressions, in fact any records that show the merits of Essiac from early use to the present . . . Sheila, I would also appreciate any information you may send me about the formula – also, if possible, assistance in obtaining herbs, knowledge about the amount used, method of brewing and any other pertinent information.'

In the follow-up letter of 26 April 1979, Dr Brusch thanked Sheila for her 'prompt and wonderful co-operation' and reported 'everything progressed smoothly' at the hearing. The fifth paragraph begins: 'You didn't happen to run into any material to help us in making the mixture, did you?'

His next letter to Sheila, dated July 1979, discusses his request for royalties as per his part of the Resperin agreement. He reports on some correspondence with Rene's niece, as executrix of Rene's estate, saying: 'She is aware of the fact that Rene and I worked together in 1959.' It is worth noting that Dr Brusch makes no mention of his having worked with Rene for 20 years, either in this letter or any of the others we have seen.

He continues:

'*Currently I am making contacts in Washington to get permission to have Essiac sent to me here at Brusch Medical. In the meantime we will work on our own formula, with your help. I am using a formula consisting of herbs given me by a friend in the Midwestern section of the USA. It has some merit but I do not know how effective it is in treating cancer. I appreciate any herbs you can send me.*'

In a letter to Mary dated 4 January 1982, Dr Brusch was still requesting herbs and instructions for making up Essiac:

'*It is very difficult for us to obtain herbs here in the States so that we can start on our project. Incidentally, any instructions or directions you can send me regarding making the mixture correctly would be sincerely appreciated.*'

In March he writes:

'*When it was not possible for me to get any Essiac after Rene's death, I happened to have a little on hand and was able to keep up the programme with . . . at reduced dosage.*'

Dr Brusch was still asking Mary for 'directions for making it' (Essiac) in July 1983 and requesting the herbs for himself to treat his cancer of the lower bowel in October 1984. A letter of 17 December 1985 mentions both Elaine Alexander and Elmer Grove of Lathrop, Missouri, 'the great herbal solution maker'. Elmer is 'very interested in working with us' on 5 August 1986, and by 14 July 1987 Dr Brusch tells Mary that

'*we are making progress, slow at times but I feel that we shall soon have the herb formula on the road. We have called it Herb Formula 1 and 5, trademark RC and CB (Rene Caisse and Charles Brusch). It is mostly "our own", plus one or two herbs which do not interfere in any way with our formula, but in fact enhance it. How happy Rene would be.*'

Sheila had met Elmer in 1979 on Long Island, following Dr Brusch's recommendation to buy a gallon of distilled turnip juice to take to a doctor in Ontario who was sick with cancer. Elmer Grove was put into a nursing home in 1991 and died from Parkinsons and Alzheimer's disease in August 1992.

Dr Brusch apparently became partners with Elaine Alexander in 1988, and was claimed to have worked exclusively with Rene Caisse for 20 years in perfecting the Essiac herbal formula. To reinforce this claim, *The Essiac Report* by Richard Thomas has reproduced a legal document signed by Dr Brusch on page 125. Paragraph 7 exactly quotes Dr Benjamin Leslie Guyatt's public statement of 1940 concerning Essiac, wrongly attributing the words to Dr Brusch over fifty years later. 'Haemorrhage has been rapidly brought under control in many difficult cases, open lesions of lip and breast responded to treatment . . . and patients with cancer of the stomach have returned to normal activity.' Dr Guyatt died of a heart attack in 1953.

Dr Brusch's health had been in a state of steady decline from 1985, evident in the ever-increasing unsteadiness of his handwriting. A postscript to a letter of 28 January 1986, typed by his wife and directed to Mary, scrawls illegibly over the page. He died on 21 October 1993 aged 85. Elaine Alexander died on 30 April 1996. The company they founded was still publishing leaflets as late as March 2000 describing Elaine as 'Today's Custodian of . . .' and discussing her in the present tense, which has proved very confusing to cancer patients prepared to put their faith in the product.

There is no evidence to prove that Dr Brusch worked with Rene for 20 years. It is generally supposed that Rene began working with him in 1958 except for the evidence of a statement made by Charles W. McClure, M.D. typed on 'Brusch Medical Center' headed paper and dated 30 November 1959 as follows:

'TO WHOM IT MAY CONCERN:

Nurse Rene M. Caisse of Bracebridge, Ontario, Canada, has for the past six months been doing Medical Research at the Brusch Medical Center, 831 Massachusetts Avenue, Cambridge, Massachusetts, under my supervision.

Very truly yours,
Signed – Charles W. McClure, M.D.
F.A.C.P. F.A.C.G.
Supervisor of Research'

If Rene had worked with Dr Brusch for the next 20 years (she died on 26 December 1978), why was there no reference to their partnership in her letters to Dr Stock at MSKCC, New York? Why would she be telling Dr Stock in a letter dated 4 August 1975 that 'you are the only person in the world that I have trusted completely' as she divulged her preciously guarded secret? And why would a working partner of 20 years' standing, who was well known in his field and headed his own medical centre in Cambridge, Massachusetts, have to write to Sheila in March 1979 to ask for reports on the MSKCC research and 'any other pertinent information'?

A handwritten note from Jane Brusch to Sheila, dated 20 January 1993, should be considered:

'Dear Sheila

Thanks for your note and information. I am infuriated over all the different things I am hearing. I can't believe that so many people are using Charlie's name and the things they are coming up with – old signatures etc – requests for peoples' records and histories – all lies. I turn all these over to our lawyer – I am dumbfounded.

Hope you are fine, Love, Jane.'

Considering Sheila's 16 years' association with Dr Brusch and his wife, and examining the evidence of the letters exchanged between them and with Mary McPherson, we must conclude that we do not believe that Rene ever gave Dr Brusch the Essiac formula. Therefore we must question any subsequent claims by people associated with Dr Brusch as having access to the original Essiac formula.

Mary's Affidavit

In reviewing the evidence of the archive material, we are satisfied that Mary McPherson remains the most credible witness to Rene's life and work. This book will refer to the basic Essiac recipe as the four-herb formula verified by Mary in her sworn affidavit of 23 December 1994, Bracebridge, Ontario, as follows:

'*6.5 cups of Burdock root (cut)*
1 pound of Sheep sorrel herb powdered
1 quarter pound of Slippery elm bark powdered
1 ounce of Turkish rhubarb root powdered
Mix these ingredients thoroughly and store in glass jar in dark dry cupboard.

Take a measuring cup, use 1 ounce of herb mixture to 32 ounces of water depending on the amount you want to make.

Boil hard for 10 minutes (covered), then turn off heat but leave sitting on warm plate overnight (covered).

In the morning heat steaming hot and let settle for a few minutes. Then strain through fine strainer into hot, sterilised bottles and sit to cool. Store in a dark, cool cupboard. Must be refrigerated when opened. When near the last when it's thick, pour into a large jar and sit in fridge overnight. Then pour off all you can without sediment.

This recipe must *be followed* exactly *as written. I use a granite (enamel) preserving kettle (10–12 qts), 8 ounce measuring cup, small funnel and fine strainer (kitchen sieve) to fill bottles.*'

THIS IS EXHIBIT 'A' TO THE AFFIDAVIT OF MARY McPHERSON SWORN THE 23rd DAY OF DECEMBER, 1994

The basic recipe – measurements and proportions

In view of the subsequent years of confusion, claims and counter-claims over the Burdock weight/volume ratio in Rene's recipe, we have opted to redefine the volume measure, preferring weight measurement for accuracy. US/Canada/UK weight measurements in pounds and ounces are identical for all practical purposes. Metric measurements are included (see *Essiac Essentials* for rationale).

6.5 US cups (24 oz/689 g) Burdock root, chopped to the size of small peas
16 oz (453 g) powdered Sheep sorrel
4 oz (113 g) powdered Slippery elm inner bark
1 oz (28.35 g) powdered Turkey rhubarb root.

This recipe produces a total of 45 oz in weight of the dried herbal mix, which could supply as many as five people taking Rene's recommended dose of 1 fl oz/30 ml of Essiac daily for over 16 months. For practical purposes, 8 oz/225 g of the herb mixture would be sufficient for one person for the minimum of one year.

Costs – trade prices/mail order prices

Organic herbs are becoming increasingly respectable and therefore valuable as marketable commodities, drawn from sources all over the world. The Essiac herbs are no exception. Distributors buy them for resale, either in bulk at the basic trade rates, with a minimum order of at least £50 to other distributors. You may be fortunate to be able to buy good-quality, organic herbs by mail order in smaller quantities to suit individual needs. We quote the most reasonable UK catalogue prices for 2000.

	Trade prices	*Per kg + tax*	
Sheep sorrel – organic	£24.67	80 g	= £1.97
Burdock root – organic	£11.16	120 g	= £1.33
Slippery elm inner bark (wild-crafted)	£17.03	20 g	= 0.34p
Turkey rhubarb root – organic	£14.10	5 g	= 0.07p

To supply one person for one year £3.71

Mail order prices for smaller quantities are proportionately higher but still represent good value for money and give you the added advantage of being able to mix the herbs yourself, retaining greater control over the even distribution of each herb in the mixture.

	Mail order prices for year 2000	Per 250 g + tax	
Sheep sorrel – organic	£12.93	80 g	= £4.13
Burdock root – organic	£6.46	120 g	= £3.10
Slippery elm inner bark (wild-crafted)	£9.40	20g	= 0.75p
Turkey rhubarb root – organic	£7.93	5g	= 0.15p

To supply one person for one year   £8.13

Supplying yourself at prices like these mean that you will only be paying the equivalent of 16p UK per week for your Essiac herbs. If you choose to buy your herbs ready mixed, you must expect to be charged for the labour, packing, postage and distribution costs involved. Whatever you choose to do, these price lists clearly indicate that Essiac can be affordable for everyone to try. No one has to be deterred from using Essiac because they cannot afford the herbs.

Packaging

Essiac is ideally packed and purchased in grocery-grade brown paper bags and stored in this packaging in a screw-top glass jar in a cool, dark, dry place until required for use. Brown paper bags that have been waxed, stuck together with toxic glue or lined with plastic to accommodate disposal of sanitary waste are not recommended as packaging for Essiac. Equally, plastic and foil packaging, while providing good protection for the herbs during product distribution, do not allow for the passage of the minute quantities of moisture natural to dried herbs and could promote mould formation over a period of prolonged storage time, especially if the packages and cartons are kept in warm conditions.

Don't waste resources

There is absolutely no need to exceed the basic dosage levels. Large doses are no more effective and waste valuable herbs. Dutch elm disease and infestation by imported insect life means that reserves of Slippery elm bark cannot be guaranteed, and demand threatens to outstrip supplies of well-harvested Sheep sorrel. Clouds Trust's work with the herbal tea has proved that Essiac works best in smaller doses, as Rene always said it would. Anything more than two fluid ounces daily as a maximum dose means overdose.

When they visited the clinic during the 1930s it must be remembered that most of the patients took a half to one fluid ounce of Essiac decoction once a week. When Rene was no longer allowed to administer the Sheep sorrel solution by injection, she recommended patients take the complete four-herb decoction in measures of 1 fl oz/30 ml once daily diluted with 2 fl oz/60 ml of hot water, to be sipped like tea, preferably before bedtime. Taking the tea at night allows for its absorption into the resting body unhindered by extraneous activity and thought. Essiac can be used as a daily tonic using ½ fl oz/15 ml of the decoction, diluted in hot water as before, with regular periods of 'time off' to maintain the impact of the body's response. In acute circumstances, 1 fl oz of the decoction can be taken twice daily for one week in every four, reverting to the single dose for the remaining three weeks. Again, an occasional week or fortnight of 'time off' can only be beneficial.

When Rene realised the doctors were administering larger doses to their patients she told Mary, 'They're just plain wasting it – it's just gone down the drain. The (body) system can only handle so much of it (Essiac) and only gets rid of a certain amount of toxins at one time.'

A question of quality

Everyone has the right to know exactly what ingredients are included in whatever medicine, remedy or supplement they are taking. Rene's legendary reticence in revealing the herbal formula died with her and can no longer be used as a valid excuse not to publish the exact content and proportion of an 'Essiac' type product. The dry herb mixture is only as viable as the herb with the shortest shelf-life, and Sheep sorrel is only viable for up to 15 months after harvesting. Making up Essiac using out-of-date, badly harvested, poorly stored and processed herbs is a complete waste of effort, money and time. The resulting sub-standard decoction either won't work or will yield a partial result, enough to make you want to buy more but insufficient to make any lasting impression.

Just because a herb is a 'herb' in a capsule or a liquid doesn't mean it automatically carries a good-quality guarantee. Don't believe you have a good product just because someone has printed the word 'herbal' on the packet. 'Certified organic' helps. Why bother spending your money feeding yourself organic foods during the day only before you go to bed to drink a brew of Essiac tea made up with herbs that could have either been subjected to an intensive farming programme or harvested from polluted sites in the wild?

The days of secrecy are past. It is vitally important for the health and well-being of those in need that manufacturers and distributors are completely open and honest about the herbs they are including in their products and which of the 'Essiac' formulae they are following. If a distributor makes any kind of change to the basic recipe and subsequently claims greater efficacy of the product, he should be prepared to provide proof of his research and results to date. 'Intuition', however strong, is fallible and not a good enough reason to make changes without giving notice to the would-be recipients.

According to Jamie Sams, Native Americans say 'when the good of the whole is placed before the good of the few, all are assured of a future filled with abundance . . . until all the People are doing well, in truth none of the People do well.' For the good of all the People, it is essential that archivists and distributors be truthful, and that all Essiac products and derivative products should be carefully prepared using certified organic herbs, with the date of manufacture stamped clearly on the package, together with complete details of content and proportion.

Chapter Two

Rene Caisse's Herbal Pharmacy

*W*e have Rene's oral and written evidence that the original recipe contained eight herbs, with Periwinkle, Red clover and Watercress in addition to the four Essiac herbs. As far as we know, she left no written evidence as to the identity of the eighth herb. Historically some Native American medicine men have been thought intentionally to omit one ingredient when describing a healing formula, believing that to reveal all their 'medicine' might give away their ability to communicate with their personal power source and jeopardise their ability to be of use to the people in times of future need. Rene always claimed to be completely unfamiliar with Native American custom. Yet she only recorded seven of the eight herbs on the paper she gave to Mary in 1977. This does not imply that Rene received the recipe directly from the medicine man, as some would have us believe, but suggests the possibility that the elderly Englishwoman may have cautioned her about the same. It is unlikely that we will ever know the truth.

Burdock, Sheep sorrel and Turkey rhubarb are all classified in Ayurvedic medicine as cooling bitters. The stabilising, grounding effect of Slippery elm is classified as sweet/neutral. As such in combination the four Essiac herbs may:

- Stimulate the immune system.
- Soothe the digestive tract.
- Stimulate the digestive system and increase energy levels.
- Relieve lung congestion by opening and clearing the respiratory tract.

- Stimulate the heart and circulatory system, cleaning the blood and relieving congestion in the lymph system.
- Reduce body heat and inflammation, reduce and neutralise acidity and toxicity, to cool and purify the blood.
- Help regulate liver functions by regulating bile production.
- Help regulate sugar metabolism and spleen function.
- Help reduce excess body fat, relieving stress on the pancreas.
- When combined, anti-tumour properties may help reduce benign and malignant tumours.

We know of four other herbs Rene used when making her kidney pills, a salve for radiation burns and a lotion for haemorrhage. Reliable witnesses have reported her using at least two more. Of these herbs, Bloodroot, Burdock, Cleavers, Gold thread, Juniper, Periwinkle, Prickly ash, Rhubarb, Sheep sorrel, Slippery elm, Red clover, Bearberry and Watercress were all growing in Ontario and would have been available to the old medicine man at the end of the nineteenth century. We have included information about Yellow dock, not because we have reliable evidence as to Rene's use of the herb but because we know that the whole herb is sometimes used as a substitute for Sheep sorrel in commercial Essiac derivatives, with possibly deleterious effect. The herbs are listed primarily in order of priority and then alphabetically where priority values are considered equal. Tables of analysis of each of the herbs can be accessed in Appendix II.

Sheep sorrel (*Rumex acetosella*, Family Polygonaceae)

Description: perennial, temperate to cold climate, soft-tissue plant (male and female), generally growing up to 18 inches (46 cm) in height, identity characterised by the narrow, arrow-shaped basal leaves.
Habitat: origin Europe, now worldwide, both Northern and Southern hemispheres.
Parts used: whole herb.

Action: astringent, cooling, diaphoretic, diuretic.
Colour in decoction: pale brown, occasionally greenish.
Solvent: water.
Commercial costing levels: medium.
Caisse pharmacopoeia: as 35% of the four-herb Essiac formula, as 100% of the Sheep sorrel decoction formula.

In order to achieve maximum potential, Essiac is dependent upon the presence and the quality of just one herb. In all her letters to Dr Stock Rene continually referred to the Sheep sorrel decoction she sent for trial to MSKCC as 'Essiac'. Without Sheep sorrel, Essiac has little value as a possibly anti-carcinogenic remedy.

Rene Caisse's 'Essiac' is well-harvested, well-stored, well-processed Sheep sorrel leaves, stems, roots and seeds collected over the season according to the growing cycle. The leaves and stems of both male and female plants are at their most potent in May and June in the Northern hemisphere, just as the first flowers are forming. The seeds are best collected in August when they are fully ripe and just about to drop. The roots should be harvested in November or December after the first frosts. Mali and Clouds Trust have spent eight consecutive seasons studying Sheep sorrel, harvesting the herb from the wild and from small organic gardens, observing the distinctive energy of the plant, the impact of its influence on the environs of its familiar habitat and its importance in the herbal decoction.

'A locally invasive tumour . . . infiltrates into surrounding, healthy tissues, sending out fingers of cells that penetrate into the mass of cells surrounding the tumour.'

Dr Grant Steen, A Conspiracy of Cells, The Basic Science of Cancer, *Plenum, 1993.*

This description could equally apply to the invasive growth pattern of Sheep sorrel in suitable conditions. Like attracts like. Like can heal like. Like cancer, Sheep sorrel thrives in acidic conditions. Like cancer, one piece of the root remaining in the soil after clearing is sufficient to regenerate its growth.

Sheep sorrel appears to choose where it wants to grow, selecting its own boundaries, either dominating an area with rampant growth or suddenly vanishing completely from apparently suitable areas for no obvious reason. Similarly, it may be impossible to rationalise an apparent failure to expand an ideal growing area in which a small, concentrated Sheep sorrel colony may be already well-established. Year after year the boundaries of the colony remain constant despite the invasive nature of the root system and regular seeding.

As an experiment, one plant colony was covered with black plastic sheeting during the winter months to encourage die-back of grasses and other unwanted plant infestation over two seasons. It was observed that as long as one small part of the plant remained visible and in contact with the elements, the root system continued to spread under the covering, sprouting up from the runners into full-sized plants ready for harvesting within three months after the sheeting was removed. The grasses and other plants were either dead or took some time to re-establish.

Sheep sorrel has also been seen to repel Ground elder, *Aegopodium podograria*, classified in the UK as a 'pernicious weed of cultivation'. In a trial planting, only one Ground elder specimen remained two seasons after the Sheep sorrel was introduced, and that specimen was growing in the shadow of a nearby Gooseberry bush, where it was observed to be protected from the energy field of the dominant Sheep sorrel colony.

A second trial involved planting Sheep sorrel around a rabbit warren where myxomatosis (an infectious disease characterised by the appearance of numerous skin tumours) was known to be endemic. The plant was previously observed to be well-established and thriving around two other rabbit warrens in separate locations where the animals were known to be healthy. The rabbits in the area of the trial planting ate all the plants within three days and consumed a complete second planting within the same time frame, suggesting the plant may have some therapeutic value for animals with this disease. The trial was not continued.

Sheila has seen Sheep sorrel growing up to three feet in height in sandy soil along major East Coast highways throughout North and South Carolina and Georgia, and in Florida south to Daytona Beach and Orlando. It may also grow wild in Arizona.

The herb grows all over Canada. In central and northern Ontario, it grows among the rocks and around the lakes, in the fields and along the roadsides but it is much smaller, growing to a height of between 12 to 18 inches. The fresh herb leaves collected from elevated, rocky sites in Canada are very slightly more pungent to taste than their European counterparts, which may be connected to the fact that the herb was growing in a particularly mineral-rich site.

Mali has found the herb growing in the black volcanic deserts in Iceland, in woodlands and heathlands in southern England, in Scotland, Ireland and Wales, in northern France, in the mountains of South Africa and in New Zealand. Sheep sorrel emigrated all over the world with the settlers from Europe, establishing itself wherever the soil was neutral to acidic, on sand, good loam and in clay. In other words, many millions of people have a possibly important remedy for cancer growing all around them, costing nothing but a little time and effort and a modest degree of understanding to effect.

THE SHEEP SORREL SOLUTION

There can be no doubt that Rene obtained her best results with Essiac during the days of the Bracebridge Clinic using a decoction of Sheep sorrel as a hypo-injection, as a topical solution, a mouthwash and as enema and douche therapies, in combination with the four-herb decoction taken orally. In her letter to Dr Stock of Sunday, 5 May 1974, 3pm from her home at 293 Hiram Street, Rene wrote:

'It took years to find out the one herb that actually worked on the growth itself. The other herbs I used to purify the blood and throw off any infection thrown off by the malignant growth as it regressed.'

The research showed Sheep sorrel, the most acidic ingredient at pH 4.5, to be the one herb that had a directly destructive effect on cancerous cells. All the initial experiments were carried out on laboratory mice:

'We found that on mice inoculated with human carcinoma, the growth regressed until it was no longer invading living tissue after nine days of "Essiac" experiments.'

Technically anyone may inject themselves with any sterile substance as long as it is not an illegal substance. Only a qualified doctor or nurse can inject another person and then only with a legally recognised, sterile substance. Rene was able to administer the Sheep sorrel decoction by injection to the patients in her clinic during the 1930s because she was a qualified nurse whose research had been encouraged by well-respected doctors of that time, including Dr Banting, who pioneered the use of insulin for treating diabetes. Early on Rene found the Sheep sorrel solution to be the only herb that could be safely injected without risk of the patient going into anaphylactic shock. Following Dr Fisher's suggestion that the treatment might be more effective if administered by injection, rather than orally, Rene wrote:

'I started eliminating one substance, then another; finally when the protein content was eliminated, I found that the ingredient which stopped the malignant growth could be given by intramuscular injection without causing the reaction that had followed my first experiments with injecting mice. However, I found the ingredients removed from the injection formula, which reduced growth of cancer were necessary to the treatment. These apparently carried off destroyed tissue and infections thrown off by the malignancy. By giving the intramuscular injection in the forearm to destroy the mass of malignant cells, and giving the medicine orally to purify the blood, I got quicker results than when the medicine was all given orally, which was my original treatment until Doctor Fisher suggested further experiments and developing an injection that could be given without reaction.'

SHEEP SORREL – ARCHIVE EVIDENCE, CANCER COMMISSION HEARINGS, 1939

Rene testified before Commissioners Wallace and Callahan at the Subcommittee hearing in Bracebridge in February 1939:

'There are a good number of patients who do not need anything but the hypodermic injection. If their general condition
is fairly good, it is unnecessary for them to take anything else
or to use anything else, but there is little or no reaction.
Occasionally I believe the treatment actually hits the seat of
the trouble or contacts the seat of trouble, there is a severe
reaction, because there are chills and fever and a slight temperature . . . but not enough to be dangerous, but for possibly
a half an hour or so and it seems that after that happens, the
patient begins to feel a decided improvement. I find that in
almost every case.'

**Commissioner Wallace questioned Rene about frequency of
the treatments:**

Q   Is it your practice to repeat the treatment several times to
    individual patients?
A   Do you mean I give them it?
Q   When do you give it to them?
A   Once a week and in some cases, twice a week. I like to
    have at least 48 hours between treatments.
Q   What length of time, generally have you continued such
    treatment?
A   Well, a good number of cases, three months. Some breast
    cases, if they are not too far advanced, will disappear in
    about six treatments.

The patients reported a variety of reaction to treatment with
the Sheep sorrel decoction. Some reported the areas around the
site of injection to be sore for a day or two after treatment,
occasionally with local reddening and irritation. It is interesting
to note Commissioner Young's asking Charles McGaughey
(Rene's lawyer and future husband) at the 4 July 1939 hearing
in Toronto:

Q   In that preparation which is used locally, is there any of
    this substance which she uses hypodermatically? Is the
    same thing used in the hypodermics as is used for these
    local applications?

Mr McGaughey: I think it is, but I will ask her and check up on it.

Mrs Elizabeth Stewart testified as a witness at both hearings. Her testimony at the Subcommittee hearing verifies her treatment by hypo-injection, oral medicine and douche therapy. Her clinic card was listed as Exhibit No. 7, she was recorded as aged 53 years at that time and her diagnosis of cancer of the uterus had been verified by Doctors Minthorne and McInnis. On page 36 of the report, Commissioner Callahan questioned Mrs Stewart to verify her condition before she attended the Bracebridge Clinic and her subsequent treatment.

Q   Were you losing weight?
A   Yes. And then I would bleed, and in the afternoons I could not eat or stoop over, or put my shoes on or take them off, I was such a size.
Q   What effect did this treatment have on you?
A   I just could not tell you, I got so much better, and all the pain left me.
Q   Did you take any douches?
A   Oh yes, I took douches and medicine and injections of stuff for cancer. When I came to Miss Caisse I could not eat and I would come in here like this (doubling over).
Q   Why? Because of the pain?
A   Pain, and I really don't know what it was; I was in such agony that I didn't know what to do.
Q   Did these injections upset you at all?
A   No, they did not.
Q   You did know you were taking them?
A   No, just on the leg where she put the needle in.

By Commissioner Wallace
Q   No chills?
A   You would get very hot.
Q   Any perspiration?
A   Yes, I would get extra hot. I got mine in the arm and I was warm.

On page 38 Commissioner Wallace questioned her about duration of treatment:

Q For about three years you have been under treatment here?
A Yes, off and on. It would not be much over a year, and maybe not run into a year.
Q How many treatments?
A Fifty-two treatments. I will tell you that is not so very many for the condition I was in, and the condition I am in today because every day I feel better.

On page 39 Commissioner Callahan asked Mrs Stewart about the present state of the tumour:

Q You said it was draining, or something to that effect. What did you mean?
A I had a discharge of this cancer.
Q Are you discharging now?
A Well, not today.
Q In the rectum, you mean?
A No, mine was from the uterus, but not today.
Q Is that continuous?
A Sometimes, and some weeks after I take a treatment, why I will have just a little bit come.
Q It seems to follow the treatment?
A Yes, it seems to follow that. Every time you take a treatment, it seems to follow that.
Q You are not menstruating at all?
A No. That passed away through three or four years ago.
Q Is it a bloody discharge?
A No, it used to be but not now. It is a kind of yellowish.
Q Any odour from it at all?
A No, not now but there used to be.
Q A bad odour?
A Yes. You could not sit in this room with it.
Q That has gone?
A Yes, it is all gone. I never had any operation.
Q No treatment?
A No.

SHEEP SORREL – ARCHIVE EVIDENCE, MSKCC, 1974–1976

Rene prepared a large stock of the decoction in ampoule form to support her research programme at the Brusch Medical Center in 1959. She kept the remaining ampoules for many years after the work with Dr Brusch was terminated in 1960, eventually sending them to MSKCC in New York for the initial laboratory trial in 1974. In a preliminary letter of 14 February 1974 to Dr Stock, Rene wrote:

'I have some ampoules I used in Boston and I know it can be used on mice or other animals as an injection . . . Mice inoculated with human carcinoma seem to get quicker results than any other type of cancer. Other types such as sarcoma take a longer series of treatments to show results. I am sure I treated all types with good results. I do not claim to have cured them all but you know I was given cases after everything medical science had to offer had been used – without results. Even then they lived longer and without *pain. After about five treatments, they stopped taking pain relievers . . . There is a lot to look for and to know how often to give injections: when a rest period would be advisable: how to stop bleeding and many other things but that can wait until you are really satisfied with your treatment of mice etc. I am taking for granted that you will. After working with patients for more than forty years, I learned many things from practical experience that not many scientists would see. Not having been taught scientifically, I had to learn the hard way.'*

Rene was more specific in her letter to Dr Stock dated 4 April 1974:

'The herb that will destroy a cancer (a malignant growth) is the dog-eared, Sheep sorrel, sometimes called sourgrass. The entire plant must be used, picked in the spring before the seeds form, then dried and powdered. One ounce of the powdered herb put in thirty ounces of pure water brought to a rolling boil and boiled for five minutes. This would reduce in the boiling to twenty-eight ounces. Turn off the heat and let stand overnight. Then pour off liquid into sterile bottles (or fill one

c.c. ampoules to keep for intramuscular injection). One ampoule should treat two mice (inoculated with human cancer) every day, (half of one c.c. to the injection). I know this all sounds crude to you but I did get results with it. Do this every day for nine days (controls for each mouse) I am sure you would get results.'

Rene appears to give conflicting advice as to how many mice should be treated per ampoule. In a letter a month later, on 10 May 1974, she wrote:

'When I was working with the doctors in Boston, I treated four mice with one ampoule. I injected it into the hip of the mouse.'

On 15 June 1974 she says:

'There is something I forgot to tell you about the "Essiac" ampoules I sent you. I kept them at room temperature over twenty years and when I used them, I stood them in warm water (the number I was to use at the time) so that they would be about blood temperature. I do not know if you will think this important or not but thought I better tell you.'

Sheila and Carroll Allen interviewed Dr Chester Stock at MSKCC, New York in February 1977. A young Dr Ralph Moss was present at the meeting, being in charge of the Public Information Office at the Cancer Center at that time. It was only then that Sheila realised MSKCC had been conducting trials solely with the Sheep sorrel decoction instead of using the complete four-herb formula. Dr Stock had no way of knowing that what Rene had sent him was not the complete formula.

During the conversation, Dr Stock referred to the earlier trials at the Brusch Medical Center in 1959–60, showing Sheila a letter revealing that some of the mice for that trial had been supplied by Dr Philip C. Merker, section head at the Walker Laboratory, MSKCC. Dr Merker had reported a physiological change in the supply animals' tumours, characterised as a tendency of the cancer cells to amalgamate and localise. This observation supported Rene's early findings in that 'Essiac' caused a secondary growth to be drawn back into the primary site, initially enlarging it before dispersal. She had written:

'In the case of cancer of the breast . . . when it becomes localised, the tumour can then be easily removed by surgery without cutting into a large area of healthy cells surrounding the growth and without danger of the tumour recurring.'

At that time, both Sloan-Kettering and the National Cancer Institute had expressed interest in these results and offered their laboratories for further testing subject to Rene providing them with the complete Essiac recipe and samples of all the herbs. In response to Rene's refusal to comply, the laboratories terminated the supply of research animals and the Brusch programme had to be halted.

Dr Stock was honest in answering Sheila's questions during the interview:

'Could the material lose its effectiveness if it was old?' asked Sheila.

'Definitely. Some ampoules we received were many years old and could deteriorate at room temperature.'

'And could human tumours react differently in comparison to animal tumours?'

'There's a decided possibility that they could,' Dr Stock replied.

(In *Cancer Biology*, 2nd edn 2000, Roger J.B. King mentions 'doubts about the relevance of animal data in human cancer' in some processes.)

There are MSKCC records of six laboratory reports on 'Essiac' experiments, the first trial conducted in 1974, a second and third in 1975, followed by three trials in 1976. *Trial one* was conducted using Rene's old ampoules made up in the 1950s previous to the Brusch clinical trials. The report of October 1974 showed no toxicity and no regressions.

Rene offered to send Dr Stock fresh supplies of 'Essiac' in January 1975:

'The reason I offered to send you more material was because I know you cannot get the entire plant. You can buy the crushed leaves but they are no good alone. I found this out when I needed so much, when treating three to six hundred people afflicted with cancer every week for eight and a half years. I do know that the whole plant is needed.'

Trial two lasted six weeks, beginning on 16 April 1975, using the freshly ground Sheep sorrel herb supplied by Rene.

At that time of year, the herb would have been part of her stock harvested the previous summer. The subsequent report indicated regressions in 'sarcoma 180' in mice treated with Sheep sorrel.

Trial three, conducted one month later, may have failed because of incorrect preparation of the material:

'*3 g of P14495 (Sheep sorrel) leaves and stem (but not roots) were ground in a mortar and the resulting suspension in 60 ml sterile water was: a) filtered through a double layer of cheesecloth, b) diluted with 120 ml water, c) placed in vials which were then refrigerated. pH = 6.1*'

[Note: Sheep sorrel in decoction should return a pH value of 4.5.]

On 4 August 1975, Rene wrote to Dr Stock in response to the lab report:

'*I am very shocked at the way your people are using the materials I sent you. The way they are preparing it for injections is an absolute waste. They might as well inject sterile water . . . They are just using leaves and stems, leaving out the roots. They are a part of Essiac and to strain it through cheesecloth destroys it. Did they ever use the ampoules I sent (60 of them)? They are what I used in Boston and got results . . . The material I sent was grown and prepared for grinding into a powder (leaves, stems and roots) and boiled. Let stand overnight (twelve hours), then poured off into sterile bottles ready for injecting. Do not strain through cheesecloth or anything else.*'

Trials four, five and six, in 1976, were delayed because of problems in the animal tumour systems. Only the January report was described 'according to prescription'. All three trials failed to repeat the positive results of trial two. The summer report was negative. It was only then that Rene learned that the mice had not been inoculated with human carcinoma. In reply to her angry letter, Dr Stock replied on 25 August 1976:

'*As you apparently wish a type of test we are not in a position to provide, nor would wish to, we will terminate our testing of Essiac. We need the test capacity for materials from others who are satisfied with our testing procedures.*'

'ACTIVE' EVIDENCE

Considering we are no longer legally permitted to inject the Sheep sorrel decoction, we have made the following recipe available on request to a small number of people, currently diagnosed with a variety of cancers, who expressed a wish to use the decoction to supplement their treatment regime. Their results have returned no adverse side effects and show increasingly encouraging action against tumour mass. They have seen the action of the Sheep sorrel decoction to be enhanced by taking the basic Essiac four-herb decoction orally once daily at bedtime. This is especially important when using the Sheep sorrel as a douche or enema. We would not use the Sheep sorrel decoction as an oral therapy, except as a mouthwash or a gargle, considering the other three herbs to act as an emollient against the immediate impact of the acidity of the herb in direct contact with stomach juices during the digestive processes.

SHEEP SORREL SOLUTION – THE RECIPE

Ingredients:
30 fl oz pure water, either filtered, distilled or bottled mineral water (pH 7).

1 fl oz sheep sorrel herb as:

- 7 g powdered leaf and stem (both male and female plants, May–June harvest)
- 1 g powdered root (November harvest, after first frosts)
- 1 g crushed seed (August harvest).

Directions:
Bring water to the boil, add powdered herb and simmer for 5 minutes.

Remove the pan from the heat, cover and allow to stand for 12 hours.

Reheat the decoction to steaming – DO NOT REBOIL!

Bottle in prepared sterilised *small* bottles, preferably 30 ml maximum. Seal immediately and well, remembering that the decoction contains no preservatives. Refrigerate as soon as the bottles have cooled.

Use:

- topically as an undiluted lotion, either to bathe the affected area once or twice daily, or to soak sterile gauze swabs to use as dressings. Change the dressings once every 24 hours;
- diluted 10 ml decoction with 20 ml water warmed to blood heat as a mouthwash once daily or as an enema or douche once every third day last thing at night on going to bed.

SHEEP SORREL SOLUTION – RECENT REPORTS
Several people have used the decoction in one of three ways, all in combination with the oral Essiac decoction and sometimes to enhance conventional cancer therapies:

- Two women applied the decoction undiluted once daily directly onto the beginnings of a recurrence of basal cell skin carcinoma. Both reported the cancer to be clear in a matter of four to six weeks.
- One lady soaked sterile gauze dressings with the undiluted decoction and applied them to a large, nodular and fungating tumour mass. She reported the hard tumour nodules at the centre of the mass to be softening and the smell to be much reduced after three weeks. The smell was gone after six weeks of treatment and the mass crusting over.
- Three women used the diluted decoction as an enema or douche to treat large metastatic tumours, secondary to ovarian cancer. The first lady reported a large inoperable tumour at the neck of womb sometime after surgery to perform a complete hysterectomy. The tumour was leaking a continual, uncomfortable, ill-smelling discharge. After three weeks of using the decoction as a douche once every third day, the lady reported her life as improved from 100 per cent unbearable to 60 per cent unbearable, and her surgeon had agreed that the discharge was cleared sufficiently to remove part of the tumour mass on compassionate grounds. The second lady reported several large inoperable tumours in the uterus and on the surface of the stomach, following the line of a previous point of entry for needle biopsy.

Within three weeks of using the decoction as a douche, the internal tumours had burst, discharging copious amounts of fluid. The patient was then considered well enough by her doctors to undertake further specialist radiotherapy treatment, something that was not an option prior to her using the decoction. The third lady has included her experience with the decoction on pages 143–6.

- A gentleman with inoperable prostate cancer has returned to work since using the combination oral/enema treatment. His full report is on pages 140–3.

- Mali's mother noticed the beginnings of her first leg ulcer shortly after her 76th birthday. A dark scab had formed over a point of previous bruising, surrounded by the characteristic purplish/red eruption common to the condition. For three days, the affected area was bathed in the four-herb Essiac decoction and covered with a dry, sterile gauze dressing. No change in condition was observed. Twelve hours after bathing the affected area with undiluted Sheep sorrel decoction, the inflammation was seen to be greatly reduced. This treatment was continued once daily. The wound was healed, with the scab drying and breaking up after five days.

Burdock (*Arctium lappa*, Family Asteraceae/ Compositae)

Description: large-leaved, downy biennial, temperate to warm climate plant, from one to two metres in height, a 'boundary and woodland clearings' plant, often found along roadsides, characterised by mature flowers forming a spiny ball with numerous hooked bracts to facilitate seed dispersal by attaching to animal fur and to clothing.

Habitat: origin Europe, emigrated with European settlers to USA and Canada.

Parts used: root and seeds.

Action: root – cleansing, detoxifying, diuretic, mildly laxative; seeds – cooling, diaphoretic, disperses congestion.

Colour in decoction: brown.
Solvents: diluted alcohol, boiling water.
Commercial costing levels: low.
Caisse pharmacopoeia: as 53% of the four-herb Essiac formula, as 21% of RMC kidney remedy formula, as approximately 4% of the RMC salve.

One of the herbs Rene asked Sheila to collect for her in 1976, the Burdock content gives Essiac its distinctive smell in preparation. Burdock is a very effective blood cleanser, providing a source of iron and inulin and useful as a detoxifying agent as the spent cancer debris is passed into the blood system. Inulin is an inverted sugar that does not employ pancreatic juices for assimilation and is recognised as having natural remedial properties in treating diabetes.

Extracts of Burdock root have been seen in experiment to show anti-bacterial and anti-fungal properties (owing to the polyolefins in the volatile oil), to lower blood sugar levels, produce diuresis (without stimulating nauseous or increased irritational side effects) and to inhibit tumour growth in animals. The viscous fibre content absorbs toxins from the bowel, lowering bowel transit time and helps to balance bacteria levels in the colon. The diuretic effect of the mucilaginous content prevents toxins from being absorbed from the digestive tract and may account for the herb's inclusion in the Essiac formula as well as the kidney formula and the salve.

As an 'active' alterative, large doses of Burdock in decoction are cautioned against in cases of severe toxicity of tissues where the immediate action of the herb in detoxifying and removing waste matter may cause a worsening rather than an improvement of symptoms. Some phtyo-oestrogenic activity has also been noted for Burdock. When Essiac is made up in the correct proportions and Rene Caisse's recommended dosage levels are adhered to, such symptomatic crises are unlikely to arise, and the proportion of any oestrogenic properties introduced by the Burdock content is thought to be minimal. The value of the herb's blood-cleansing and detoxicant effects should outweigh any unproven, deleterious action of what is thought to be a small element of an unspecified phyto-oestrogen.

Evidence from studies on the effects of phyto-oestrogens is varied with no obvious guidelines emerging. Research has yet to be carried out over a long enough period of time to be conclusive, with the possible exception of Red clover (see page 62). In view of the effect of the Burdock content in Essiac, it should be remembered that the original recipe was formulated exclusively for a woman with breast cancer. Breast and uterine cancers were routinely successfully treated at the Bracebridge Clinic, the most conclusive evidence for the value of 'Essiac' as a remedy for the 'female' cancers being shown when the oral decoction and the Sheep sorrel decoction therapies were used in combination. With reference to the six case-history books available to us from the Bracebridge archive:

- *Book one* lists 16 patients of whom four had possibly hormone-related cancers – x1 uterine, x1 prostate, x1 uterine/breast, x1 cervix;
- *Book two* lists 16 patients of whom six had possibly hormone-related cancers – x2 breast, x2 uterine, x1 cervix, x1 ovarian;
- *Book three* lists 20 patients of whom eight had possibly hormone-related cancers – x2 cervix, x3 prostate, x2 breast, x1 uterine;
- *Book four* lists 12 patients of whom four had possibly hormone-related cancers – x1 uterine, x3 breast;
- *Book five* lists 18 patients of whom six had possibly hormone-related cancers – x3 breast, x2 uterus, x1 cervix;
- *Book six* lists 16 patients of whom two had possibly hormone-related cancers – x1 breast, x1 prostate.

Unfortunately, if Rene's uncorrected recipe, as given to Mary, is currently commercially in use, such a product would increase the proportion of the Burdock in the respective product to 80 per cent of the formula instead of the recommended maximum 53 per cent. Such exaggeration in proportion not only substantially reduces the possibly anti-carcinogenic effects of the Sheep sorrel content in the remedy but increases the chances of both symptomatic crisis and possibly adverse phyto-oestrogenic activity occurring. This could be particularly significant if the recipient is taking several large daily doses of 'Essiac' in the mistaken belief that if a little helps, a lot helps more. This course of action may not be recommended for some breast and uterine cancers. It should be noted that since Burdock is less expensive to produce than Sheep sorrel, the Burdock-prominent, incorrect formula is a more attractive marketing proposition to cost-conscious distributors.

Slippery elm (*Ulmus rubra* – formerly *fulva*, Family Ulmaceae)

Description: a temperate climate, deciduous tree, growing up to 60 feet (20 metres) in height, characterised by large, rough, irregularly serrated leaves, downy young twigs and deeply furrowed, grey, sometimes reddish bark.
Habitat: native to eastern states, USA/Canada.
Parts used: inner bark only.
Action: demulcent, emollient, nutritive.
Colour in decoction: red.
Solvent: water.
Commercial costing levels: moderate.
Caisse pharmacopoeia: as 9% of the four-herb Essiac formula, as 11% of the kidney remedy formula, as approximately 4% of the salve.

Traditionally a Native American remedy, the coarse outer bark lacks the healing power of the fine inner bark. Externally the tree presents as a rough, 'hairy' specimen, the leaves and young 'stems' being contact-toxic to some people and capable of producing severe to extremely severe symptoms of contact dermatitis as in itching, burning and raised and reddened skin. The pollen from the dense clusters of flowers has also been noted as toxic to some people.

Internally, Slippery elm has healing, mucilaginous, non-toxic qualities, its presence in the four-herb decoction both complementing the influence of Burdock and considerably increasing the action of Essiac's vital mucilage content. Both herbs are also included in the kidney remedy and the RMC salve and may have similar activity in both formulae. Like Burdock, Slippery elm derives such properties from polysaccharides, which have a slippery effect, are mild-tasting and swell in contact with water to produce a slimy, protective coating for any exposed surface. These protective properties are particularly useful for the lining of the digestive tract, soothing and reducing symptoms of irritation, and are invaluable in the treatment of digestive disorders. Polysaccharides, by reflexive action, have been seen as palliative in disorders of the bronchial and urinary ducts. Mucilaginous plants have the ability to retain heat and have been used for centuries to make warm compresses. In addition to mucilage, Slippery elm bark contains twin crystals of calcium oxalate, and decoctions of the herb can be drunk hourly to coat the throat and allow the tannins to congeal and discharge excess mucus.

Slippery elm enjoys the same benefits of viscous fibre as Burdock, but the demulcent action of Slippery elm is said to be negated when prescribed in capsule form for respiratory treatment. It is similarly negated in capsule form for Essiac. We would go so far as to say that we consider the actions of all four Essiac herbs to be considerably reduced when presented in capsule form as the quality of the remedy depends upon the strength and unique blending achievable only in decoction.

Unlike the other three herbs, Slippery elm is becoming an endangered species, having endured years of decimation by Dutch elm disease and more recently the ravages of a Chinese beetle mistakenly imported into the Eastern states. Harvesting effectively kills each tree, and as demand increases for the herb, suitable substitute products may have to be considered. In his book *Planetary Herbology*, first published in 1988, Dr Michael Tierra refers to *Fremontia californica*, Family Tiliaceae, a tree native to California, as having properties and uses nearly identical to the predominantly East Coast native, Slippery elm. *Fremontia californica* is said to grow abundantly in the southern Sierra Nevada region. In Europe, Iceland moss (*Cetraria islandica*, Family Parmeliaceae), a lichen recorded as showing some antibiotic action, is less nutritive than Slippery elm but possesses similar mucilaginous properties and might be considered as a viable replacement. As far as we know, no trials for substituting either of these herbs for Slippery elm in the Essiac decoction have yet been carried out.

Most of the world supply of Slippery elm bark comes from the USA where the crop is routinely fumigated with ethylene oxide, a known carcinogen. The use of ethylene oxide has been banned for more than eight years in the UK and is banned in Europe. However, it is still legal in the USA, and products treated with ethylene oxide can be exported to Europe. Mention this to your supplier before you pay for your herbs.

Turkey rhubarb (*Rheum palmatum*, Family Polygonaceae)

Description: a perennial, temperate to cool climate, large ornamental plant, bisexual, characterised by large palmate leaves coarsely hairy on the veins underneath, on stout stalks in basal clumps surrounding the large flowering stem, which can grow up to eight feet in height. Not to be confused with the smaller, edible garden rhubarb.
Habitat: native to western China and Tibet, now found in suitable regions worldwide.
Parts used: root only.
Action: astringent, cooling, diuretic, laxative.
Colour in decoction: orange-brown.
Solvent: water.
Commercial costing levels: moderate.
Caisse pharmacopoeia: as 2% of the four-herb Essiac formula.

Turkey rhubarb is listed as a sister plant to Sheep sorrel, and, while it does not exhibit the range of possibly anti-carcinogenic properties of the latter, it is invaluable for its cleansing properties and ability to relieve pain and reduce fever and inflammation. Unlike Sheep sorrel, ingesting any part of Turkey rhubarb leaves or stalks causes a severe toxic effect and must be avoided at all costs. The six-year-old, golden-brown roots, which yield a distinctive golden-brown powder, are the only part of the plant used medicinally.

Recorded in a Chinese herbal dating back two thousand years, Turkey rhubarb root has a complex chemistry most easily divided into the two basic categories of anthraglycosides and tannins. In small doses (as in Essiac), Turkey rhubarb has more of the tannin, astringent effect, acting as a valuable stimulant to digestion and a tonic, increasing the appetite, stimulating salivary and gastric juices and cleansing the liver by stimulating the gall duct to expel accumulated bile toxins. Large doses induce the purgative anthraquinone effect, a cathartic effect caused by glycosides. Some anthraquinone derivatives have a dilating effect on the colon muscle, while others cause contraction. Depending on the size of the dose and the way in which it is given, Turkey rhubarb is effective as a regulating agent for both constipation (anthraquinones) and diarrhoea (tannins).

Dr Edward Shook reported the powdered rhubarb as being used in colonial British East Africa during the nineteenth century as a treatment for acute bacillary dysentery, in doses as '30 grains every 2 or 3 hours until the rhubarb appears in the stools. After a few doses, the stools become less frequent. Haemorrhage ceases and straining and other symptoms of acute, general poisoning which characterise the disease, rapidly disappears.'

Rheum palmatum is the preferred rhubarb representative for inclusion in the Essiac decoction as being more medicinally potent, distinct from its close relative, *Rheum officinale*, commonly known as Indian rhubarb. Rene listed 'indian rhubarb' on the paper she gave to Mary in 1977, which Mary duly corrected to 'turkish' rhubarb. This listing may provide a useful indication of which formula a commercial distributor might be following, as indicated on the relevant packaging. It may be important when estimating the possibility of the product carrying a greater Burdock proportion than is considered appropriate to the Essiac recipe.

Rene Caisse's kidney remedy

We believe that Rene developed her recipe for the kidney pills during the latter part of the 1930s, primarily to treat men with prostate and related urinary problems. She never considered taking out a patent on the Essiac formula because she knew she would have to reveal the recipe. She had no such reservations about the recipe for the kidney pills and, following the suggestion of Health Minister Harold Kirby, she made formal application for a patent with the assistance of Mr Egerton R. Case, Specialist in Patents and Trade Marks, in July 1940. The patent for the kidney pills was granted on 5 August 1941 to Rene M. Caisse-McGaughey of 249, McIntyre Street, North Bay, Ontario for 'an alleged new and useful improvement in Compositions of Matter for Treatment of Diseases of the Urinary Organs and Processes of Compounding Same'. The patent was granted initially for a period of 17 years, after which time Rene was obliged to renew annually until she was granted a life-time patent. This patent was officially withdrawn in 1976. She applied for the trademark registration 'R.M.C.' on 28 February 1942, to be granted on 16 November that same year.

Initially she made up the pills herself until the manufacturing was taken over by a pharmaceutical company. The tablets were on sale in all the local drug stores from the 1940s up to 1976 when the patent was suddenly cancelled. In 1976, 50 tablets were selling for $1.75 CAN.

THE PATENT (29 JULY 1940)

We reproduce the complete patent specification as detailed by Rene Caisse, including the wording of the flyer accompanying each package and two of the five testimonies from successfully treated patients as submitted with the application.

The invention relates to a composition of matter for the treatment of diseases of the urinary organs and a process of compounding the same, and the object of the invention is to utilise the combined ingredients when absorbed into the system, to secure a reaction on the urinary organs so that when a retention of the flow of the urine is experienced, the flow will be gradually increased to normal. When there is a frequency of the flow it will be gradually reduced until it is normal, while at the same time the action of the bowels will be gently accelerated. The result is that the health of the patient is gradually improved owing to the positive removal of waste matter through the urinary tract and the bowels which are caused to co-ordinate their functional activities . . . The most beneficial results were found to flow from the use of the composition in affections of the prostate gland and enlargement or inflammation of any of the urinary organs.

The ingredients are first thoroughly ground to a powder and then thoroughly mixed in this form to ensure that the properties of the compound will be the same throughout. Then water at atmospheric temperature is added to the powdered mass and mixed to form a paste. Pills are formed from this mass containing preferably five grains each.

The composition consists of the following ingredients: prickly ash berries, juniper berries, burdock root, uva ursi and slippery elm bark.

In making up a quantity of the composition, the ingredients are used in the following proportions:

2 pounds of powdered prickly ash berries
1 pound of powdered juniper berries
1 pound of powdered burdock root
2 ounces of uva ursi
one half pound of powdered slippery elm bark

The composition is administered in doses of from one to four pills daily. The patient is advised to drink at least six glasses of water each day.

The composition gradually assists nature to restore to functional co-ordination of the urinary organs and the bowels to remove bodily waste accumulated during the lack of functional co-ordination between them.

Rene published the following directions for patients taking the pills:

R.M.C. Remedies:

Do you tire easily?

Are you subject to frequent urination?

Do you spend restless nights having to get up?

Do you have backache?

Do you feel lifeless?

Any of these symptoms may indicate that the kidneys are not functioning properly.

The kidneys help in the elimination of the waste products of digestion. If your kidneys are not functioning properly, these destructive substances may be retained and absorbed by the system and may cause other disturbances.

R.M.C. Kidney Pills were compounded to relieve these conditions.

R.M.C. Kidney Pills are efficient and are especially beneficial to men in and beyond middle life. After middle life one may need such medicine. Take two pills a day, one in the morning on an empty stomach and one before retiring, followed in each case by a glass full of warm water until your condition improves. Then it is advisable to reduce the quantity to one pill a day each morning immediately after rising. The action of the tablets are (sic) greatly accelerated by drinking from six to eight glasses of water a day.

These tablets are purely herbal, a mild laxative and harmless to young and old alike.

Young and old alike are benefited by the use of these tablets.

Directions for use

One tablet in the morning directly on rising with a glass of warm water.

One tablet on retiring with a glass of warm water.

Continue until noting improvement when dosage may be reduced to one tablet each morning. The action of the tablets are (sic) greatly accelerated by drinking six to eight glasses of water daily.

TESTIMONIES
The testimonies of five gentlemen patients signed under oath verifying the efficacy of the tablets were included with the petition for the patent. We have included two testimonies:

HORACE PIERPOINT OF WEST FERRIS, NIPISSING, a Railway employee:

1. I have had kidney and bladder trouble for the last six years.

2. I have treated with four different doctors during that time but have obtained little relief and my condition became worse and I was obliged to quit work for weeks at a time.

3. My back was very weak and I have been suffering severe pain and obliged to urinate at night as many as four or five times.

4. I started taking Mrs McGaughey's red kidney pills a month ago and have felt greatly relieved. The swelling in my hands and legs has gone down; I do not have to urinate more than once at night. The urine has become clear and I felt greatly improved in health.

5. My greatest help has been the ease with which I can now urinate, whereas a month ago I suffered terribly with restricted and very painful flow.

Sworn December 27th 1940 in North Bay

JOHN THORNBURY, OF ELDON, VICTORIA, a Farmer:

1. I am sixty years of age.

2. My kidneys started to bother me two years ago. My doctor told me my Prostate gland was enlarged and my kidneys affected. I used several bottles of medicine prescribed by him but I only obtained temporary relief and my condition became worse. I had severe pains in my back and would have to urinate as often as six times at night.

3. I started taking Mrs McGaughey's red pills for kidneys in June 1940 and have been taking them regularly since then and at present in less quantities.

4. In two weeks I began to get considerable relief. My pain disappeared entirely, my urine became clear and the flow normal, and it is only once in a week or two that I have to urinate at night, and then only once.

5. I find that my Prostate gland does not bother me now and my health is greatly improved.

Sworn December 22nd 1940 in Bracebridge

Some years after Rene's death, Mary McPherson updated the recipe to include making the kidney remedy in capsule form.

RENE CAISSE'S KIDNEY REMEDY – MARY'S MODIFIED VERSION

Formerly known as RMC Kidney tablets

Ingredients: 2 lb Prickly ash berries, powdered; 1 lb Juniper berries, powdered; 1 lb Burdock root, powdered; 8 ounces Slippery elm powdered inner bark; 2 ounces Uva ursi (Bearberries) powdered.

- Mix the four powdered herbs together thoroughly, kneading well before blending them in a grinding machine. Empty the powdered mixture into a large bowl.
- Use number 2 sized capsules for this remedy. These can be purchased from a local drug store for about $30 CAN per thousand.
- Fill each capsule by scooping the mixture into the larger half of the capsule, then pushing this part against the inside part of the bowl to ensure that the mixture is packed firmly. Repeat this action until the capsule seems to be full and firm to the touch.
- Continue to fill each capsule until the mixture of powdered herbs is all used up.
- Take one capsule on rising in the morning with a cup of warm water and a second capsule with a cup of warm water just before bedtime. Continue until improvement is noted; then dosage may be reduced to one capsule

daily. The action of these capsules is greatly accelerated by drinking 6–8 glasses of water daily.

Note: These capsules may be used for kidney, prostate and urinary problems. When good quality Prickly ash berries are not available, substitute powdered Prickly ash bark.

DOSAGE NOTES

Taken in tablet or capsule form in small doses, the uncooked herbal compound would be relatively mild in action. Mali experimented by making a decoction using 1 fl oz of the herb mixture to 30 fl oz of water, boiling for 10 minutes and leaving to stand overnight before bottling. The resulting mixture was red, pungent and strong. Mali and three others tried one dose of 15 ml of the decoction diluted in 30 ml water with the following results:

- Mali – felt an almost immediate sense of cramping in her right side around the area of a deformed (since birth) ureter duct from the kidney to the bladder. The cramping sensation continued for half an hour until she drank several glassfuls of water, and the area remained sensitive until the following morning. At the same time, a mild, chronic, hay fever-type, summer sinus blockage disappeared almost immediately for four hours. Mali repeated the experiment once more a few days later with identical results. She did not continue the trial.
- Volunteer two – an elderly lady, felt a similar cramping around the bladder, which was not relieved until she drank some water. The area remained sensitive for some hours. The trial was not repeated.
- Volunteer three – drank several glasses of water immediately after taking the diluted decoction. She felt no sensation of cramping or discomfort. The trial was not repeated.
- Volunteer four – experimented taking the decoction once a day for a week using 30 ml decoction to 60 ml water to treat a chronic bladder infection of some years' standing

with related pain, a burning sensation and bleeding when urinating. She drank as much water as she could comfortably manage during this period. Initially she experienced cramping and a constant pressure to pass water. She also experienced two bouts of diarrhoea, the first within three hours of taking the decoction and the second two hours later. By the second day the problem was stabilising. The pain was gone, there was no more diarrhoea and no more pressure to pass water. By the end of the week the condition was clear and the treatment was discontinued.

While we are aware that the remedy can be effective in capsule form, we do not recommend using the herbs as a decoction, given the possible effects of the irritant elements of the Juniper content being greatly magnified at this level. The case histories included with the patent application indicate a dosage period of not longer than six months. We would recommend that the capsules are best taken for shorter periods of time, for not more than six weeks at any one time, with a break of perhaps two weeks to a month between.

Prickly ash (*Zanthoxylum americanum*, Northern prickly ash/*Z. clavaherculis*, Southern prickly ash, Family Rutaceae. Note: *Zanthoxylum* is sometimes spelled as *Xanthoxylem*)

Description: a small tree with pinnate leaves and alternate branches covered in sharp prickles, the deep blue/black berries grow in clusters at the top of the branches.
Habitat: native to North America, from Canada to Virginia and west to the Mississippi.
Parts used: berries and bark.
Action: analgesic, stimulant, diaphoretic, promotes saliva.
Colour in decoction: red.
Solvents: boiling water, dilute alcohol.
Commercial costing levels: moderate.
Caisse pharmacopoeia: as 43% in the RMC kidney remedy.

Z. americanum bark includes several coumarins including *zanthyletin*. *Z. clavaherculis* lacks the coumarins. The two Prickly ash barks are not completely identical but have been seen to be very similar in their activity, yielding a large amount of ash, 12 per cent or more on combustion. The dried bark was listed in the *US Pharmacopoeia* as a treatment for rheumatism from 1820 to 1926.

The berries are higher in volatile oils and are considered stronger in action than the bark. The berries of both species are thought to be equally similar in activity and were listed in the *US National Formulary* from 1916 to 1947 for having anti-spasmodic, stimulant and anti-rheumatic properties.

Prickly ash is considered a useful remedy for chronic inflammatory disorders where deficient circulation is indicated. When swallowed, the bark produces a sense of heat in the stomach, stimulating arterial action and a tendency to perspire. The berries and bark can be used as a tonic in debilitated conditions of the stomach and digestive organs, for flatulence and diarrhoea, and are used in colic, cramp and cholera, in fever, ague, lethargy and for cold hand and foot complaints arising from poor circulation. Native Americans pulverised the root or the bark to treat toothache and were known to use a decoction of the same to treat venereal disease. Acting as a counter-irritant, the decoction may be applied on compresses and has also been used as a remedy to stimulate or hasten menstruation in women. There are no reports of adverse side effects.

In considering Prickly ash as a possible anti-cancer remedy, isolated enzophenanthridene alkaloids have been reported to be destructive to cancer cells (L.J. Hartwell, *Lloydia*, 34, 1971, 103). No other evidence is currently available.

Prickly ash berries are important in the Caisse pharmacopoeia in that they constitute almost 44 per cent of the kidney remedy formula. Prickly ash was one of the herbs we know Rene was still using in 1976 because she asked Sheila to collect it for her. Prickly ash shares the possibility with two others of having been the eighth herb in the original eight-herb recipe, simply because: a) it features so predominantly in the kidney formula as to suggest that Rene was long familiar with its properties, and b) it should have been readily available to the old medicine man in northern Ontario at the end of the nineteenth century. Rene may have included Prickly ash berries in the kidney remedy on account of their anti-inflammatory properties and to stimulate both the blood supply to the urinary organs and urinary flow. She chose to use the more potent berries when available in preference to the bark. There is no evidence to suggest Rene may have ever included Prickly ash as part of the oral Essiac formula.

Juniper (*Juniperus communis,* Family Coniferae)

Description: an evergreen shrub, growing either flat on sand or rock in colonies up to 12 metres across or upright reaching approximately one metre in height; the leaves open in whorls of three, with a white stripe down the middle of the leaf, strongly scented, flowers appearing in May and the fleshy, dark blue to purple/black berries maturing at the end of the second year after flowering.

Habitat: many varieties worldwide, native in three indistinct varieties to North America, mostly on dry, rocky areas in poor soil, found in Canada, south to New Jersey, west to Nebraska and in the mountains of New Mexico.

Parts used: the dry, ripe berries.

Action: carminative, stomachic, stimulant, fumigant, diuretic, expectorant, disinfectant, digestive, antiseptic.

Colour in decoction: pale red–brown.

Solvent: boiling water/alcohol.

Commercial costing levels: moderate.

Caisse pharmacopoeia: as 21% in the RMC kidney remedy.

Juniper berries were listed in the 1868 list of Canadian medical plants (*Can. Pharm. J.* 6, 1868, 83–5). Taken in small doses, as in the RMC kidney pills, the berries should act as an antiseptic and serve to reduce irritation, acting as a gentle diuretic and stimulant. In contrast, if taken in large quantities or made into a strong decoction, Juniper berries have been seen to cause irritation of the urinary passages. Juniper is listed as an unsafe drug in the USA and should not be to be used as a remedy for more than six consecutive weeks.

The constituents in the volatile oil make the herb a potent diuretic. As such, the berries can be valuable in treating acute inflammatory conditions and are best used in conjunction with other herbs to increase the effectiveness of more powerful diuretics in treating fluid retention problems rather than taken alone. The action of the herb may have a deleterious effect on the kidneys when used consistently over a period of time, and the berries should never be taken during pregnancy as they are known to stimulate uterine contractions, possibly precipitating abortion. The distilled oil from the plant should never be used internally.

Native Americans regarded Juniper as a 'hot' remedy and used almost every part of the plant for 'cold' disorders. They ate the berries and the inner bark to prevent starvation. Some tribes dried the berries and ground them up to bake into cakes. Others ground the roasted Juniper berries for use as a substitute for coffee. Both berries and bark were used as a remedy for coughs and colds and sore throats. The leaves and stems were boiled to make an astringent tea in British Colombia. Juniper berries are also used to flavour gin. Gin (juniper and alcohol) and tonic (water and quinine) was taken on a daily basis in nineteenth-century British colonial India as an anti-malarial remedy. When considering Juniper as a fumigant, S. Kneip, author of *My Water Cure* (1897), advised:

'Those who are nursing patients with serious illnesses such as Scarlet fever, small pox, typhus, cholera, etc, and are exposed to contagion by raising, carrying, or serving a patient, or by speaking with him, should always chew a few juniper berries (6 to 10 a day). They give a pleasant taste in the mouth and are of good service to the digestion; they burn up as it were, the harmful miasms, exhalations, when these seek to enter through the mouth or nostrils.'

The decoction was recommended as a spray for fumigating a room used by a patient with an infectious disease. Juniper has also been used as an effective anti-parasitic to kill worms in children and adults, and has a reputation in folk medicine as an anti-cancer remedy. More recent studies have identified anti-tumour activity in animals, together with strong cytotoxic activity in cell culture against HeLa cancer cells (see page 84). Anti-viral activity in cell culture against influenza virus A2 and herpes simplex virus 1 and 11 as well as anti-bacterial activity against several human disease-promoting pathogens have been observed.

Rene was still using a tincture of Juniper in 1977, Carole Allen having observed a bottle in the fridge in the house on Hiram Street, although whether Rene was using the tincture for patients or for herself is unclear. She suffered from fluid retention for many years and may have used the Juniper tincture alongside the Essiac to increase diuretic action. As far as we know, she left no instructions regarding this. The Juniper content was undoubtedly the irritant factor identified in the previously mentioned voluntary trials using a decoction of the kidney remedy, although this irritant quality should be placated by the mucilaginous properties of the Burdock and Slippery elm content in the remedy.

Bearberry (*Arctostaphylos uva-ursi*, Family Ericaceae)

Description: a perennial, temperate to cool climate, small shrub with many short and woody branching stems, growing in dense colonies; small, leathery green leaves, upper surface dark, shining green, lower surface paler, young leaves fringed with short hairs which drop off during the drying process; waxy flowers appear at the end of the branches May/June, and bright red, smooth, glossy berries ripen that same year.
Habitat: northern latitudes of the Northern hemisphere and high mountains of Europe, America and Asia. Common in Scotland, northwest Ireland, Canada and the US as far south as New Jersey and Wisconsin.
Parts used: leaves.

Action: marked diuretic effect, astringent, soothing, anti-viral, anti-fungal, anti-plaque, enhances cytotoxic activity.
Colour in decoction: pale green.
Solvents: alcohol, water.
Commercial costing levels: low.
Caisse pharmacopoeia: as 3% of the RMC kidney formula.

Bearberry leaves have a long history of use as a soothing diuretic. Some old herbals and pharmacopoeias still list Bearberry under *Arbutus uva-ursi*, as the plant was formerly assigned to the Arbutus genus. The Black bearberry (*Arctostaphylos alpina*), found in northern Scotland, represents the only other British species assigned to the Arctostaphylos genus. Cowberry leaves (*Vaccinium Vitis-idoea*) and box leaves (*Buxus sempervirens*) are occasionally used as substitutes but do not have the same activities and values as Bearberry.

Native American women used the herb for menstrual remedies and to promote labour contractions. Bearberry mixed with honey, pollen and various other herbs made a popular longevity elixir. European herbalists have long considered the herb to be of great value in treating bladder and kidney disorders, and in strengthening and toning the urinary passages. Inflammations of the urinary tract, as in acute cystitis, were commonly treated with a decoction of Bearberry leaves, which turned the patient's urine a greenish colour during the course of the treatment.

Bearberry's diuretic action and harmless change of urine colour have been found to be due to the presence of the glucoside arbutin, which the body converts to hydroquinone, a urinary disinfectant (Martindale), exerting an antiseptic effect on contact with the urinary mucous membranes. This action has been found to be particularly effective with alkaline urine (as when the patient follows a vegetarian diet – D. Fiohne, *Planta Med*. 18, 1, 1970). The allantoin content in the leaves soothes and accelerates the repair of irritated tissue and does not cause gastric irritation. Allantoin has the quality of being extremely and immediately diffusable throughout the body and will contact deep tissues from external application. Present-day user-friendly shaving balms advertise an allantoin content to soothe razor-damaged skin.

Acting in combination with Juniper as an enhanced diuretic in the kidney formula, Bearberry's allantoin strengthens the activity of the soothing and healing mucilaginous properties of the Burdock and Slippery elm content while supporting the anti-inflammatory and circulatory stimulant properties of Prickly ash. There is no evidence to suggest Bearberry was ever part of the oral Essiac formula.

Balsam of Peru (*Myroxylon pereirae*, Family Leguminosae)

Description: a large and beautiful tree with a straight, smooth trunk yielding a valuable, mahogany-type wood; heavily scented flowers.
Habitat: the forests of San Salvador in Central America.
Parts used: an oleoresinous liquid, i.e. resin mixed with volatile oil and gum.
Action: antiseptic, anti-parasitic, expectorant, stimulant.
Colour in decoction: insoluble in water.
Solvent: alcohol.
Commercial costing levels: moderate.
Caisse pharmacopoeia: as approximately 5% of RMC salve for radiation burns.

Every part of the tree, including the fruit and the leaves, is capable of producing a rich, sweet, resinous juice. The bark contains a gum resin, which changes from yellow to amber to dark brown. The beans contain coumarin, and the husks have an extremely acrid bitter resin and a volatile oil. The tree is productive after five or six years of growth and can continue to yield for up to 30 years. The extraction process produces three grades of balsam in that time.

Balsam of Peru is warm and aromatic, being hotter and more stimulating than Balsam of Copaiba, which is sometimes sold as a substitute. It is commonly used externally to treat skin disorders, including parasitic infestation, and is considered useful for rheumatic pain. The benzoic acid content makes Balsam of Peru equally a good local antiseptic in small doses and a local irritant in large doses, exhibiting the same qualities when used both externally and internally. It is also used in soap manufacturing because it makes a soft and fragrant creamy lather, soothing for chapped hands.

Undoubtedly familiar with Balsam of Peru as an antiseptic wound dressing, Rene included it as the key constituent in her salve for radiation burns. We do not know for certain if her recipe for the salve was one of her own making or something she had used during her nursing days in the Ontario hospitals. We have no personal experience of the salve's efficacy in treating radiation burns. The recipe for the salve is included as recorded by Mary McPherson.

R.M.C. SALVE
3/4 lb (12 oz) lamb fat (organic)
1 fluid oz Balsam of Peru
4 fluid oz Castor oil
4 fluid oz glycerine
1 tbs Slippery elm bark
1 tbs powdered Burdock root

Method:
Put Balsam of Peru in a bottle and pour in 4 oz Castor oil. Let stand for one week before pouring off and mixing with melted lamb fat. Add all remaining ingredients and heat in a low oven or double boiler for two hours. Strain and beat the mixture at intervals while cooling until it is thick and looks like cold, whipped cream. Pour into small jars. Rene used this salve for radiation burns.

Mary says that the salve is messy and takes time to make but the end result is worth the effort. A little goes a long way, and it makes the skin so soft you can use it on your face. It is good for all skin complaints, especially stress-related eczema, and takes the soreness out of burns.

Note: when Mali made the salve, 12 oz of lamb fat rendered and filtered down to 8 fl oz, and the completed recipe filled 36 x 15 ml jars. The salve showed an immediate effect on a subsequent burn, taking away the stinging and redness and leaving the area unmarked within 24 hours. The clearing up after making the salve was the messiest part of the whole five-hour procedure, needing some fairly concentrated detergent to melt the grease from the cooking utensils.

Bloodroot (*Sanguinaria candensis*, Family Papaveraceae)

Description: a perennial, temperate to warm climate plant with palmate leaves, six to eight inches long; a single, shining white, waxy flower with bright yellow stamens is produced early in spring on a 20 cm reddish stalk enfolded by large, half-opened leaves, presenting as prominently veined and palmate, blue–green leaves, 15–25 cm long when fully open after flowering.
Habitat: native to eastern and midwestern North America, preferring open, deciduous woodland.
Parts used: dried rhizome and root, whole plant.
Action: anti-pyretic, antiseptic, cardio-active, cathartic, emetic, mucous expectorant, spasmolytic, stimulant, topical irritant. *Contraindicated for general use.*
Colour in decoction: red, diluting to yellow.
Solvents: alcohol, water.
Commercial costing levels: medium.
Caisse pharmacopoeia: as an ingredient in RMC solution for ulcers and ulcerated wounds, percentage uncertain.

Bloodroot was classified as unsafe by the US Food and Drug Administration in March 1977. It is similar to Foxglove (*Digitalis*) and Ipecacuanha in action and has been found to be toxic in anything more than very small, controlled therapeutic doses. The decoction tastes particularly nasty to drink, causing almost immediate nausea and vomiting in most people and leaving an unpleasant and persistent after-taste in the mouth.

Other side effects include a burning sensation in the stomach, intense thirst, faintness and vertigo with related adversely affected vision.

The high dose of astringent tannic acids in Bloodroot derive from the tormentil content in a herb which is known to be emetic and purgative in large doses, stimulant, diaphoretic and expectorant in small doses. Do not use this herb internally as an enema or a douche as Bloodroot is known to damage sensitive membranes. For the same reason the powdered root must not be inhaled, although it was once recommended as a snuff for treating nasal polyps.

Native Americans used Bloodroot as a facial dye, as a tea for treating rheumatism and as a remedy for ringworm. Topical preparations including sanguinarine have been useful in treating eczema, possibly contributing a mild, local anaesthetic effect. Extracts of Bloodroot included in mouthwashes and toothpaste are thought to help prevent cavities and destroy plaque. Warts have been treated with the fresh juice, and possible anti-bacterial and anti-cancer activity has been reported (A. Leung, op. cit.). As a folk remedy, Bloodroot has been applied to fungal skin growths, visible cancers and ulcers.

In 1977, Dr David Walde, who was researching the formula, reported some of the 'Essiac' vials Rene gave him for use on his patients were discoloured with an orange–red substance, which he believes could have been Bloodroot. It could have also been due to the presence of Cleavers root, another herb he identified in some of the preparations Rene sent him.

Rene has left us no written evidence of dosage levels or percentages in proportion in formulae. Aware that she occasionally used Bloodroot in her nursing practice, we have included information about the herb, but we do not advocate its general use as part of the Essiac treatment.

THE RMC SOLUTION FOR ULCERS

Mary wrote out the following recipe for Sheila, the only evidence we have for Rene's using Bloodroot as part of a remedy:

RMC solution

As used for cleansing wounds and to stop bleeding.

1 oz Sheep sorrel (fluid ounce)
1 oz Bloodroot (same)
32 oz water.

Boil together for 10 minutes, let stand until cool, strain and bottle. Use 2 tablespoons to a cup of warm water to kill odours and heal.

Mary says Rene used this solution on ulcers from varicose veins and to bathe affected cancers, leaving to dry and repeating three or four times each day. However, we do question the accuracy of quantity of Bloodroot (classified as a toxic herb) as recommended in this recipe and would not use it ourselves. We consider the reported results using Sheep sorrel alone in decoction sufficient verification for the efficacy of the remedy. *Bloodroot should never be used internally*.

Cleavers (*Galium aparine*, Family Rubiaceae)

Description: a herbaceous, temperate to cool climate annual plant with slender, angular stems and leaves arranged in whorls, both covered with little hooked barbs to enable the plant to attach itself to passing objects or adjacent shrubs, often forming matted masses over the same on reaching sufficient light to sustain growth; flowers appearing May to September are small and greenish-white, followed by bristled seedheads, which scatter by clinging to the coats of passing animals.
Habitat: abundant in Europe and North America as a hedgerow weed.
Parts used: leaves, stems, seeds.
Action: blood purifying, diuretic, alterative, aperient, tonic.
Colour in decoction: brown.
Solvent: water – do not boil.
Commercial costing levels: low.
Caisse pharmacopoeia: included, proportions and uses uncertain.

Known as a 'lymphatic' herb and traditionally seen as a rather powerful diuretic, Cleavers has been recommended as a remedy for promoting urinary secretion and the action of the urinary organs, particularly in cases of kidney or bladder stones blocking the urinary ducts. It is also used to treat a variety of skin diseases, with the crushed herb applied as a poultice directly on sores and blisters, and has a curative reputation as a remedy for cancer, particularly cancers of the lymphatic system. The roots contain a red dye that appears to tinge red the bones of birds that habitually feed on the plant.

Cleavers could be considered as a possible candidate for the eighth herb in the original recipe. Dr Walde detected the aroma of the plant in a trial sample, and his finding a leaf in the brew confirmed this, suggesting Rene may have used that plant when her stocks of the usual herbs were running low. We do not know which type of cancer he was intending to treat with the sample. As a possibly anti-cancer herb, Rene may have used Cleavers to substitute Sheep sorrel in part. However, we must point out that Rene did not work willingly with Dr Walde, and it is possible that she may have included a small proportion of the plant to fool him into thinking that Cleavers was part of the formula. We do not consider the evidence for its possible inclusion in the Essiac formula to be strong enough to experiment with the herb in this way ourselves.

Gold thread (*Coptis groenlandica*, indistinguishable from *Coptis trifolia*, Family Ranunculaceae)

Description: a small, cool climate perennial plant with obdurate, evergreen leaves growing in tufts with yellow scales at the base, found as creeping, many-branched and matted colonies of slender, bright golden yellow rhizomes in dark swamps or damp, sandy places on relatively infertile acidic soils and peatlands – in Ontario, Gold thread favours a habitat under or near Black spruce trees; the solitary yellow flowers appear from May to July depending on altitude.

Habitat: Greenland, Iceland, North America and Asia.

Parts used: the dried rhizome as roots, stems, leaves.
Action: astringent, tonic, stimulant, a bitter digestive.
Colour in decoction: yellow.
Solvents: boiling water, dilute alcohol.
Commercial costing levels: very high.
Caisse pharmacopoeia: included, proportions unknown.

Gold thread resembles Gentian and Quassia in its properties
and Golden seal (*Hydrastis canadensis*) in action. Lacking either
tannic or gallic acids, Gold thread's activity depends on berberine,
a bitter alkaloid with anti-bacterial and anti-protozoal properties,
which acts as a sedative to the central nervous system. It is
associated with coptine, which may act as a stimulant to the
autonomic nervous system, as in regulating involuntary action of
the heart, intestines and the glands. *The herb is contraindicated
in pregnancy and in cases of high blood pressure.*

Native Americans used Gold thread as a yellow dye and as
a mouthwash. They chewed the roots to treat mouth sores and
made a tea from the roots as a general tonic and to treat
indigestion. Gold thread was the '*tissavoyane jaune*' of the
French Canadians who used the roots and leaves to dye flax,
skins and wool yellow. As a folk remedy the herb is taken to
promote digestion by improving the appetite and acting as a
general stimulant to the system, either administered alone or in
combination with other herbs.

Sheila met an elderly gentleman in Bracebridge who had
known Rene Caisse during the 1930s. He lived in Minett,
Ontario and had been driving his brother to Bracebridge once a
week for treatment at the Cancer Clinic. Rene mentioned to him
that she was looking for a supply of the Gold thread herb
because she knew it grew in the swampy areas around Minett at
that time. The man was so grateful for her treating his brother
that he collected and dried enough of the herb to fill a large bag.
When he gave it to Rene he was surprised to see her begin to cry.

'Oh, what a wonderful gift you have brought to me,' she
said. 'It is exactly what I've been needing to use on some of my
patients.'

It may be concluded by Rene's reaction to her gift that Gold thread was obviously important in her pharmacopoeia and, given its possibly catalytic properties when used in conjunction with other herbs in a prescribed formula, could be considered as our third, and perhaps the strongest candidate for the eighth herb in the original recipe. Native American medicine men were known to use the herb as a tonic to stimulate the system after prolonged illness and, like Golden seal, Gold thread has a traditional reputation as an impetus to positively stimulate the activity of other herbs in an otherwise relatively inactive prescription. These herbs are especially useful when treating toxic, inflammatory and congestive conditions.

Mali had been looking for the herb in Iceland and trying to find to someone who knew where it was growing while she was in Canada. Resigned to returning to England empty-handed, she met a lady on the bus from Bracebridge to Toronto, one of those chance meetings that don't happen by chance. They were talking about cancer and Essiac, passing the time on a two-hour bus ride, when the lady suddenly said, 'My mother-in-law drank Gold thread tea for years. It grew where our old house used to be, long yellow roots you had to pull up out of the ground. Mother-in-law drank the tea for strength and she could still arm-wrestle her grandkids in her eighties.'

We do not know exactly how Rene was using the herb. We know that some patients were treated with the oral four-herb decoction alone. We know that others were treated with Sheep sorrel as a hypo-injectable therapy in conjunction with a Burdock, Slippery elm and Turkey rhubarb decoction as an oral treatment. Some may have been treated with both the four-herb decoction and the hypo-injection simultaneously, depending upon their individual needs. It is possible that Rene may have made use of Gold thread's catalytic properties in either the three-herb or the four-herb oral decoctions for certain patients, and the herb may well have been included to act as a highly beneficial and potent catalyst in the original eight-herb recipe.

Periwinkle (*Vinca major, vinca minor*, Family Apocynaceae)

Description: a perennial, trailing, 'ground-cover' plant with glossy, dark green leaves and blue, purple or occasionally white flowers only producing seed in its native southern Europe; otherwise spreading via extensive root systems. *Vinca major* has larger, egg-shaped leaves with minutely fringed margins. *Vinca minor* leaves are much smaller and their margins are not fringed.
Habitat: worldwide.
Parts used: leaves and stems.
Action: anti-haemorrhagic, astringent, tonic.
Colour in decoction: pale yellow–green.
Solvents: water, alcohol.
Commercial costing levels: low.
Caisse pharmacopoeia: included in the original eight-herb formula, proportions uncertain.

Greater periwinkle is the species more generally employed in herbal medicine as a laxative and a gargle and to treat haemorrhage and unusually heavy menstruation in women. As an ointment, the herb is taken for piles and inflammatory conditions of the skin. Lesser periwinkle is used in homeopathy to make a tincture to treat haemorrhages. Both species of periwinkle are used for their 'binding properties' in natural medicine. Periwinkle tea as an infusion is considered a good remedy for relieving mucoid congestion in the intestines and lungs and to treat diarrhoea.

The Madagascan periwinkle (*Catharanthus roseus*) is assigned to a separate genus, Lochmera, and is now classified as an important medicinal source of the anti-leukaemic drugs vinblastine and vincristine. Vincristine is used for childhood leukaemias, vinblastine for certain types of Hodgkin's disease; it may cause a marked decrease in white blood cell count. Madagascan periwinkle cannot be safely recommended as a herbal remedy as its side effects can cause potentially life-threatening complications.

Vinca major and *Vinca minor* (Greater and Lesser periwinkle) are chemically and pharmacologically quite different from *Catharanthus*. *Vinca major* and *minor* are also different chemically although both species contain astringent tannins and alkaloid vincamine, which is said to improve blood flow to the brain and to have a contracting effect on uterine muscle.

Dr Brusch reported to Sheila that Rene had told him Periwinkle was included in the original eight-herb recipe when they worked together in 1959, and we have her written evidence as to its inclusion in the paper given to Mary McPherson in 1977. We should point out, however, that Periwinkle was one of the herbs Rene discarded from the formula during her early research, and we see no valid reason for its inclusion in the remedy today.

Red clover (*Trifolium pratense*, Family Leguminoseae)

Description: a short-lived, warm to temperate climate perennial plant up to 60 cm in height, flowering from May to November with pairs of trifoliate leaves surrounding each globular, red–purple flowerhead.
Habitat: native to Europe, now worldwide.
Parts used: flowerheads.
Action: alterative, anti-spasmodic, deobstruent, diuretic, expectorant, sedative.
Colour in decoction: pale red–brown.
Solvents: boiling water, alcohol.
Commercial costing levels: low.
Caisse pharmacopoeia: included in the original eight-herb formula, proportions unknown.

In common with many other members of the Leguminoseae family, Red clover absorbs nitrogen from the air and transforms it into soil-enriching compounds, making it a useful soil enhancer and natural fertiliser when grown and ploughed back into the earth. Clover is a favourite animal forage in the wild for bears, deer, elk, game birds and songbirds. Native Americans ate clover leaves, stems and roots, and made bread from the dried flowers to nourish the people during famine times. They were familiar with the herb as a treatment for cancer, and generally used the whole plant as a medicine, externally in ointments for external skin conditions and internally as a tea to treat skin diseases.

Although Red clover is still considered as a possible cancer remedy today, it is also a source of naturally occurring plant oestrogen and potent in that its oestrogenic properties may be more easily absorbed and utilised by the body than any synthetic counterpart. Coumestrol, present in large quantities in Red clover, is a powerful phyto-oestrogen, the effects of which are possibly accumulative, even in small quantities, when taken regularly over a period of time. A past president of the British Veterinary Association told Mali about a report from New Zealand where sheep were failing to become pregnant while grazing on pasture heavily infested with clover. A similar story was reported as long ago as 1946 in Australia (*J. Dept. Agric. West. Aust.* 23, 1946, 1–12). In both cases, the clover was acting as a contraceptive, similar in action to the 'Pill' women have been using with varying long-term results since the 1960s.

As such Red clover presents a dichotomy of possible activity in that extracted isoflavone biochanin A is said to be a potent carcinogen inhibitor while coumestrol, daldzein and genistein have recently been shown to exhibit the potential to induce chromosomal abnormalities in human blood cells (*Arch. Toxicol.* 73, 1999, 50–4). This implies that in some cases the herb may serve to stimulate rather than suppress the production of mutant cells.

To date research is inconclusive on the true effects of the use of phyto-oestrogens in treating oestrogen-dependent cancers, and Red clover may not be recommended as a remedy for such cancers. In this instance the questionable benefits of the oestrogenic properties of the herb may outweigh the apparent benefit of its anti-carcinogenic activity when treating hormone-related cancers. We have no way of knowing whether the original English woman patient was cured of an oestrogen-dependent cancer.

When Rene and her home were under police protection after the *Homemakers* article was published in 1977, the old bunch of Red clover hanging up near her furnace regularly fooled those visitors who did make it through the front door into believing they were seeing one of the 'miracle' herbs. Rene admitted more than once that Red clover was in the original eight-herb recipe but, because of its high protein content, it was one of the first of the original eight herbs she and Dr Fisher decided to discard when working together to develop what would become the Essiac formula.

It might be wise for anyone with an oestrogen-dependent cancer to be cautious when using an 'Essiac' derivative product that includes Red clover. A combination of the known phyto-oestrogenic properties of Red clover with the possibly similar, weaker properties of Burdock could have a deleterious effect if used in large quantities over a prolonged period.

Watercress (*Rorippa nasturtium-aquaticum*, Family Cruciferae)

Description: a perennial plant with branching underwater stems 30 cm–100 cm long, with rounded, dark green leaves and flowers growing above the water level; small white flowers appear between April and October.
Habitat: native to Europe, emigrated to North America with the settlers, growing most freely in shallow, running water.
Parts used: leaves and root.
Action: blood purifying, stimulant, diuretic, expectorant, laxative, a nutritive tonic.
Colour in decoction: pale green.
Solvent: water.
Commercial costing levels: low.
Caisse pharmacopoeia: included in the original eight-herb recipe, proportions uncertain.

Rich in minerals and vitamins C and E, Watercress is a valued food source and a traditional herbal remedy for treating fluid retention and mucus in the lungs, acting as a metabolic stimulant (particularly for bile metabolism); it is considered a useful remedy for indigestion and stomach gas. Native Americans used Watercress for liver and kidney trouble and to dissolve kidney stones.

The herb is a valuable source of iron in the diet and exceptionally high in sulphur and mustard oil glycosides, which are primarily locally irritant to membranes and therefore useful as poultices to increase blood flow and to treat inflammation. Mustard oil glycosides can depress thyroid function when eaten in quantity.

We know Rene was still using Watercress occasionally alongside the four-herb formula into the 1970s, employing the herb cautiously and selectively but not habitually. It may have been one of her 'back-up' herbs when other stocks were low. Again, Watercress was one of the herbs she discarded during her concentrated research programme in the 1920s, and we know of no valid reason to disturb the synergy of the four-herb Essiac formula by the inclusion of this herb now, believing it to be far more useful as a fresh food source of minerals and vitamins in the daily diet.

Yellow dock (*Rumex crispus*, Family Polygonaceae)

Description: an invasive, perennial plant up to 150 cm in height with narrow, lance-shaped leaves crisped or curled at the edges; flowering June to October in dense, greenish to red whorls; the roots are thick and yellow when cleaned and peeled.
Habitat: origin Europe, now worldwide as a weed.
Parts used: root and rhizome.
Action: astringent, detoxicant, blood-purifying, alterative, affecting the circulatory and digestive systems, the liver and gall bladder.
Colour in decoction: red–brown.

Solvents: alcohol, water.
Commercial costing levels: moderate.
Caisse pharmacopoeia: not noted, no evidence either written or oral.

Yellow dock leaves have a high oxalic acid content and are not generally recommended for internal use, being most familiar to us as an instant source of relief from the itching and burning after touching Stinging nettle leaves. In decoction, the root, stem and leaves are markedly less acidic than Sheep sorrel, returning pH 6.5 against Sheep sorrel's pH 4.5. Native Americans used the crushed leaves of the herb to draw pus out of boils and applied the pulverised root to cuts to prevent infection. The herb's value was quickly recognised by Native American medicine men, especially when treating jaundice and skin disorders.

The root decoction was a popular remedy for a variety of ailments in the nineteenth century and listed in the *US Pharmacopoeia* from 1863 to 1905. Later *The Dispensary of the United States* declared the herb to have no real value. However, modern herbalists recognise the roots as being rich in a complex mixture of anthraquinones, anthraquinone glycosides and tannins based on emodin and chrysophenic acid, and comparable in activity to Rhubarb, for which Yellow dock is sometimes substituted.

We have included information on Yellow dock because the roots have been noted as having an unusual ability to absorb whatever iron is available in the soil, making the herb a bioavailable source of potentially high doses of iron and an effective treatment for anaemia. Michael Moore says Yellow dock liberates iron stored in the liver. This is possibly an important factor in considering a report from the USA where a few people taking Essiac have experienced a marked elevation in iron levels in their blood, causing some concern to themselves and to their doctors.

Burdock contributes the greatest proportion of the iron content in the four-herb formula, with trace amounts from Sheep sorrel and Turkey rhubarb. There are no records, either from the Bracebridge Clinic days or from present-day Essiac users in the UK, as having reported unusually high iron levels in their blood when using the herbal remedy at the correct dosage levels. However, it is known that some 'Essiac' distributors use Yellow dock as a cheaper and more alkaline substitute for Sheep sorrel, particularly in the USA. We suggest that anyone taking Essiac or a derivative who is showing high iron levels in their blood may be inadvertently using incorrect herbs at unnecessarily high dosage rates. In such cases, it may be useful either to change suppliers or to purchase the individual herbs and make up the decoction yourself at home.

Chapter Three

What is Cancer?

'A patient has the right to information about treatment.'
Royal Marsden Nursing Manual, UK, 1999

*T*his statement is repeated 84 times in this standard teach-textbook for nurses, a book easily obtained from distributors around the world and stocked in bookshops in the UK. But do we understand the information when it is offered? And with a cancer diagnosis ringing in our ears, are we in a suitably attentive state to hear what is being said?

Nurses are instructed to 'evaluate the patient's knowledge of the medication/treatment offered. If this knowledge appears to be faulty or incorrect, offer an explanation of the use, action, dose and potential side effects of the drug or drugs involved.' This is to ensure that we, as the 'patient', understand the procedure and give our 'valid consent'.

Most of us don't have a clue. To the untrained, a hospital is a place where we go with a greater or lesser degree of fear, either to sit in a waiting room or to be put to bed, there to receive a share of a variety of treatments on offer, most of which are invasive, many are terrifying and few are clearly understood. It is well known that doctors and nurses make notoriously bad patients – have you ever wondered why?

Ignorance can be bliss, but long term, a little basic knowledge at the outset goes a long way to better understanding. It helps to know what is going on in your body when you are given a cancer diagnosis, and you must understand the nature of the treatment you are undertaking when you sign the consent forms. 'Valid consent' should mean exactly what it says, consent with full knowledge and agreement. So many people, Mali included, say with hindsight 'I would have done it differently if I had known then what I know now.'

So what is cancer?

Cancer is a multi-cellular disease natural to a multi-cellular being – you. Your body is an ordered mass combination of approximately 75 trillion cells divided into thousands of different and interdependent cell types. During your daily living process your body routinely produces a minute percentage of abnormal cells. As you are reading this page, whether or not you have had a cancer diagnosis, your immune system is routinely mopping up these abnormal cells, any one of which could become cancerous if the right conditions are allowed to prevail.

Cancer isn't selective. No one body is particularly singled out to get cancer, and cancer doesn't just happen to 'everyone else'. We all have cancer one way or another. We are all multi-cellular beings, and we are all capable of producing cancerous cells. In 1985, Fallon and Hawtrey reported the results of tests on the adrenal glands of 169 normal but aborted human foetuses, which showed each of the glands examined contained nests of cells usually classified as neuroblastoma cells and capable of producing a highly malignant tumour of the nervous system common to the adrenal gland. The authors concluded that the spontaneous regression of neuroblastoma cells seems to be a normal feature of foetal development.

In other words, it is possible that every one of us has already had cancer and dealt with it while still in the womb.

How healthy cells work

Normal cells consist of:

- A nucleus, containing chromosomes, which consist of tightly bundled strings of genes, each of which carries tiny molecule beads of coded information (DNA).

- Cytoplasm, surrounding the nucleus and comprised of tiny, energy-producing particles and millions of different molecules necessary to produce hormones, enzymes and energy to maintain your body. Vitamins and minerals are key component chemicals in cytoplasm.
- The cell wall membrane, a thin, oily layer made up of fatty lipids surrounding the cytoplasm that allows the free passage of nutrients and cell-produced chemicals between the cell and the bloodstream.

Normal cells are able to grow and divide throughout the normal life span. That is to say, they are able to replicate themselves to replace cells lost during the normal course of the body processes and to heal the body after injury. As yet it is impossible to observe the complete life cycle of healthy cells since cells are microscopic and not generally available for individual examination in a living human body. Not one of us is going to lay on an operating table for as many days or weeks as it takes while scientists watch the exact life cycle of a small clump of cells forming, maturing and dying in whatever of our organs they have chosen to study.

However, living cells are routinely extracted during surgery (as in taking tissue samples for biopsy) and can be grown in a dish in a laboratory. Under such conditions scientists have recognised that normal cells are limited to the number of divisions they undergo, less in the cells taken from older people than younger ones. Normal cells are controlled by tightly regulated growth factors and retain their resemblance to the particular tissue from where they were originally obtained. In the laboratory they are seen to grow in a uniform manner until they cover the bottom of the culture dish. They stop growing when they encounter one another. In other words, normal cells are contact-inhibited and are programmed to stop growing when they have attained the shape and structure necessary to maintain the characteristics of whatever organ they represent.

How cancer cells work

Cancerous cells in the laboratory grow in a very different way from normal cells. Often they bear no resemblance to the tissue type from where the samples were originally taken. Under favourable conditions in a culture dish, cancer cells appear to be no longer contact-inhibited and go on growing and dividing until they form a piled-up mass in the bottom of the dish. Occasionally some cells will detach themselves from the mass and form separate clumps of cancerous cells floating in the culture medium, similar to a cancer metastasis.

If the culture dish was a pliable membrane instead of a rigid glass or plastic structure, theoretically the cells would continue to grow, feeding on the culture medium and distorting the contours of the dish until the membrane was completely full. As in a tumour, the atmosphere inside this membrane would be increasingly lacking in oxygen and nutrients and would be essentially hostile to cell growth. While the outer cells at the edges of the membrane would continue to grow, many of the cancer cells furthest away from the culture medium at the centre of the growth would starve and die, forming the characteristic necrotic mass seen in large, well-established tumours. The few strong cells that survive this hostile environment will become increasingly capable of further mutation and resistance to treatment. Normal cells never behave like this.

What causes cancer

There are eight principal causes:

- Hereditary and hormonal factors.
- Exposure to chemicals, including some drugs used for cancer chemotherapy.
- Exposure to the carcinogens in tobacco smoke.
- Exposure to certain viruses.
- Dietary factors.
- Exposure to radiation, including sunlight, X-rays and radiotherapy treatment.

- Regular and prolonged alcohol consumption, especially in combination with tobacco use.
- Physical trauma, resulting in local deoxygenation of tissue, as in the formation of scar tissue.

Various cancers have certain potential causes in common. Cancers of the colon, rectum and stomach are thought to be connected with dietary causes, particularly with low fibre/high fat diets. A high dietary intake of fat and also eating a large proportion of dairy foods (as in products from cows) are thought to possibly stimulate breast, ovarian, endometrium and prostate cancers. Exposure to certain herbicides and DDT molecules may increase risk of breast cancers, and dry cleaning chemicals (Perc) have been linked to increases in the incidence of oesophageal and bladder cancers and leukaemia. Alcohol consumption is thought to exacerbate cancers of the colon, larynx, liver, mouth, oesophagus, pharynx and rectum. Tobacco smoke carcinogens have been linked to bladder, kidney, lung, mouth, nose and throat, oesophageal and pancreatic cancers, while genetically induced chromosomal changes in the cells have been indicated as a potential cause of the colorectal cancers, chronic myelogenous leukaemia, brain tumours and the skin cancers, including malignant melanoma. The increase in use of domestic pesticides has been linked to a rise in soft tissue and brain cancers in children.

How cancer begins

Cancer begins when a single abnormal cell avoids being mopped up by the immune system and begins to divide, producing two identical daughter cells that are equally capable of growth and division while escaping the vigilance of the immune system. These cells undergo a typical cell life-cycle pattern except that they are liable to increasing mutation as they develop, typically losing up to one-third of all their original genetic information as they attain full malignancy. Even then there may be insufficient oxygen and nutrients within the cell mass to maintain active growth, and the tumour may go into a state of dormancy that may last for years without achieving fully active malignancy status as a tumour mass in the lifetime of the person involved.

So don't think that all pre-cancerous cell masses always progress into cancer. They don't. They can stay dormant or they can regress and disperse. We have all probably had pre-cancerous cell masses at some time in our lives that have dispersed and disappeared, not noticed, not diagnosed and not feared. It is only when a tumour has been allowed to evolve sufficiently to stimulate the growth of new blood vessels within the mass that the resulting blood-born resurgence of oxygen and nutrients stimulates renewed active growth. This new growth speeds up the rate of cell mutation and promotes the formation of invasive and possibly metastatic growth. If we have been casual about cancer prevention before this happens, now we will have to start pay a great deal of attention to getting well.

Initiators and promotors

The instigation of the development of our single abnormal cell into a cancer cell depends upon an 'initiator' event and a 'promotor' event occurring in that order.

- The **initiator** can be an entirely random event involving high- or low-key exposure to any one of the carcinogenic agents to allow for the further mutation of a routinely abnormal cell.
- The **promotor** can be apparently completely unrelated to the initiator, involving exposure to a carcinogenic agent or agents, perhaps over a long period of time. This allows for an increase in the speed of division and mutation of the abnormal cells into pre-cancerous masses of cells before progressing to full-scale malignancy.

A possible example of this process could involve a typical 25-year-old male who smokes socially, perhaps only five to 10 cigarettes a week. He drinks an average of six cups of coffee a day and a glass of beer or wine with a meal most evenings, occasionally followed by a glass of spirits. At weekends he drinks and smokes more frequently. He eats meat usually once every day, sometimes twice. He exercises mainly at weekends when he remembers.

He has a routine chest X-ray as part of a medical examination before taking up an offer of a new job in another country. The radiologist is not quite satisfied with the quality of the image and asks for a retake. The second image is satisfactory, nothing abnormal is diagnosed and our subject passes the medical. Unknown to him and the medical team, a routinely produced abnormal cell was exposed to radiation twice within two hours while he was being X-rayed. The DNA in this 'initiator' cell has been damaged enough for the cell to by-pass the immune system and, while it may remain dormant for many years, our man's lifestyle inadvertently acts as a 'promotor', slowly weakening the immune system until the abnormal cell re-enters the cell cycle and begins to divide and mutate. Our subject goes to see his doctor at around 50 years of age with various symptoms, and a diagnosis of cancer of the lungs or of the oesophagus results.

How do tumours metastasise?

Metastatic or secondary tumours occur when malignant cells gain access to a free passage-way through the blood circulatory system or the lymphatic system. They break away from the primary tumour to be carried along with the blood or lymph fluids until they attach themselves to a nutrient-rich site (for them) and begin to establish a colony of mutant cells that may or may not evolve into a secondary tumour. A classic example involves mutant cells from a primary bowel cancer escaping through the hepatic portal vein and setting up a secondary colony in the liver, which is already weakened after months of processing toxic chemotherapy.

However, you should realise that most metastatic tumour cells die during this process. Only a very few of the most aggressive cells have the possibility of survival, and then they only succeed in forming a secondary tumour if the immune system has been sufficiently weakened to allow the right conditions for abnormal growth to continue.

Defining your diagnosis – what does it mean?

Having asserted your right to access your notes, it is highly likely that you may find yourself presented with a diagnosis scripted in a medical and biochemical terminology that is almost completely unfathomable. Doctors habitually use complicated biochemical language in order to classify the growth disorder of the cells in a tumour, words which usually mean absolutely nothing to the person who has the tumour.

You may find any one of four different words attached to your 'cells' in your diagnosis:

- **Hyperplasia** Hyperplastic cells are not expected to become malignant.
- **Dysplasia** Dysplastic cells are considered to have the possibility of progressing to malignancy over a long period of time.
- **Metaplasia** Metaplastic cells are more unusual and are considered to lead to highly malignant forms of cancer
- **Anaplasia** Anaplastic cells divide at a higher rate than normal cells and are expected to show a greater degree of structural abnormality. Anaplasia is common to most cancers, and doctors often base their prognosis on the degree of anaplasia present in a particular tumour.

The word 'differentiation' usually comes into it as well. Well-differentiated cancer cells still look something like the original tissue cells on site of the tumour. For example, well-differentiated liver tumour cells will still bear some resemblance to normal liver cells, while poorly differentiated cancer cells will be so abnormal (anaplastic) that it is difficult to identify the original tissue type.

Mali was presented with the following information when she asked to see her husband's pathological report after a brain tumour was diagnosed. She read it through several times and went completely blank. How does a collection of words like this relate to the body of the living, breathing person you know and love?

Using Electron photo-micrographs to help define the tumour cell type using biopsy fragments extracted from the tumour during surgery, the study revealed 'a poorly differentiated, highly cellular tumour composed of spindly cells with fairly abundant fibrillar cytoplasm. The cells are reminiscent of spongioblasts. Occasional giant nuclear forms are seen. Rare cells are binucleated. Irregularly shaped cells with enlarged, irregular nuclei are seen. The cytoplasm contains intermediate filaments, some lysomal structures and polyribosomes.'

Diagnosis: Posterior Fossa Brain Tissue: Glioblastoma Multiforme.

Translated, this report describes a grade four brain tumour at an advanced stage of cell mutation. The spindly cells 'reminiscent of spongioblasts' still bear a vague resemblance to the embryonic cells typical of the connective tissue of the central nervous system that certain brain tumours are known to develop from. Some cells have a double nucleus, and others have severely abnormal nuclei, bearing no resemblance to normal brain cells. No metastasis is noted as the tumour was a primary tumour. Secondary brain tumours usually grow only after the primary tumour has been removed by surgery.

All the abnormal cells listed in this report are capable of dying. All cancer cells are capable of dying. They can only live if they are continually supplied with nutrients. The so-called immortal cancer cells are only immortal because they are being fed. Starve them and they will die.

Conventional cancer therapies

It would be absurd to dismiss almost a century of research into cancer – with varying degrees of both ethical practice and success – exclusively in favour of the complementary therapies, most of which have yet to be properly tested. In an ideal world, both the conventional and selected complementary therapies would work alongside each other, and doctors and their patients would discuss all the options available when selecting suitable therapies to treat the cancer in question. It can be an ideal world if enough of us know enough to be satisfied with nothing less.

Conventionally, most people are offered variations on the three basic therapies in cancer treatment, ranging from fairly standard tried and tested procedures to others that are purely experimental. Surgery can be radical or used therapeutically to relieve blockage or pressure of a tumour on vital organs when it is not possible to fully remove the growth and when quality of life may be enhanced by surgical procedure. Chemotherapy and radiotherapy work best when used to treat rapidly growing cells that are well supplied with oxygen. If a tumour mass is slow-growing and supporting a lot of dead and dormant cells, neither chemotherapy nor radiotherapy are likely to be successful in the long term.

Surgery

'Tumours get angry when they are cut' (Dr J.M. Hunter Holmes McQuire Veteran's Administration Hospital, Richmond, VA, July 1993, to Mali).

This kind of statement is not easily forgotten, particularly when the patient in question has just come round from a third operation in as many weeks.

So why do we cut cancer? Because surgery is still the primary cancer therapy, usually followed by chemotherapy or radiotherapy or both. Surgery alone is most likely to be successful if the tumour is found to be sufficiently encapsulated to be removed whole. If a tumour has to be cut into and removed in pieces, a single surviving cancerous cell left behind after surgery will be sufficient to regenerate future growth. In *Cancer of the Head and Neck* (1989) E.L. Barnes noted cancer cells as being present in the washings from surgical wounds in 10 to 15 per cent of cases. If these figures are typical of cancer surgery in general, the surgeon should only consider operating on a non-invasive, non-metastic primary tumour that is easily located and capable of being removed in one whole section, together with sufficient surrounding tissue that will not cause unnecessary post-operative damage to the patient.

Surgery is often recommended simply to obtain a biopsy sample to verify a doctor's diagnosis in order to justify the expense of treating a patient with cancer. It is not unknown for cancer patients to undergo potentially life-threatening procedures simply to extract tissue samples for examination in the laboratory. Mali's husband Greg was in theatre for eight and a half hours for a biopsy sample to be removed from the brain tumour to verify a diagnosis already considered to be 90 per cent certain from MRI scans. The resulting brain damage from such invasive surgery took months of precious time to recover from.

In 1993, in *A Conspiracy of Cells, The Basic Science of Cancer*, Dr Grant Steen points out that 'about fifty percent of all cancer patients probably have occult (hidden) metastases at the time of diagnosis and treatment'. Seven years later, in his *Cancer Biology*, Professor R.J.B. King notes that 'it has been estimated that, at first detection, seventy percent of cancers have spread elsewhere in the body and are not amenable to surgical removal'.

This means the successful outcome of surgery and the associated therapies should be carefully questioned and considered before consent is given, especially as there is some evidence of an essential energy connection between primary tumours and metastic secondary tumours, however far apart they are established in the body. B. Fisher *et al.* reported tests on mice in 1989 that showed metastasised cells in secondary tumours accelerating their growth rate following surgery to remove the primary tumour.

Chemotherapy

Cancer chemotherapies are classified as 'cytotoxic' drugs. *Cyto* means 'cell' and *toxic* means 'lethal', which literally translates as drugs that kill cells, both healthy and malignant cells. Many cytotoxic drugs have been shown to be capable of causing mutation of normal cells, and some are thought to be capable of producing abnormalities in a developing foetus and in cancerous cells when administered to human or animal patients. In other words, some of the drugs that you are being given to kill the cancer are actually capable of causing cancer. Professor King writes 'that patients who receive chemotherapy have a ten-fold increased risk of developing leukaemia . . . an acceptable risk'. This doesn't mean to say that everyone who has chemotherapy is automatically going to need further treatment for leukaemia, but it does question the possible long-term effects of the treatment.

Handling these drugs doesn't help pharmacists and nurses either. Referring to the *Manual of Clinical Nursing Procedures*, nursing staff have reported the following symptoms: headaches, nausea, dizziness, lightheadedness, coughing, hair loss, skin irritation and generally feeling unwell. Given that these occupational risks are listed as being hazardous and of increasing concern to hospital administration authorities, it is not unreasonable to suggest there must be some concern for those patients who are elected to be on the receiving end of such treatment. And as both normal and cancer cells are more prone to mutation in older people, it might be advisable to question the value of aggressive chemotherapy when treating people over 60 years of age.

Many cytotoxic drugs are only tolerable if they are rapidly diluted in fast-flowing blood, as when they are injected directly into a vein. If they are spilled undiluted onto the skin or leaked into surface and surrounding tissues, for example, if the needle isn't properly inserted into the vein, these chemicals can cause severe damage to healthy tissue, including necrosis, the irreversible death of tissue. Such spillages must be treated immediately to avoid pain, possible physical defects, the need for hospitalisation for plastic surgery and delays to further treatment as well as all the mental and emotional stress that goes with it. Commonly used chemotherapies capable of producing tissue necrosis include: carmustine in concentrated solution, dacarbazine in concentrated solution, dactinomycin, daunorubicin, doxorubicin, epirubicin, idarubicin, mithramycin, mitomycin C, mustine, streptozocin, vindesine and vinblastine, and vincristine, as derived from the Madagascan periwinkle (see page 61).

It is worth knowing that some non-cytotoxic drugs commonly in use are also capable of causing severe tissue damage if inadequately administered. These include: amphotericin, acyclovir, ganciclovir, phenytoin, potassium chloride, hypertonic solutions of sodium bicarbonate if greater than 5 per cent and vancomycin. If you have been prescribed any of these drugs, take care to read the instructions carefully and follow them equally as carefully.

Other cytotoxic drugs are produced in tablet or capsule form. It doesn't make them less hazardous to handle, just easier to administer. Nurses and pharmacists dispensing these drugs are instructed to use 'non-touch' techniques at all stages of handling the drugs. Risk is reduced when tablets are coated or when 'there is no free powder visible'. So don't think about quietly reducing your chemotherapy by breaking your tablets/capsules, and don't attempt to crush a tablet to make it easier to swallow.

In the same way that bacteria become immune to antibiotics, tumour cells become immune to chemotherapy if a drug is given at low levels over a period of time. Combination doses of two or more different chemotherapies given in intensive, short-term doses are considered to be the most effective in killing cancer cells. At the same time they are equally effective in killing and damaging healthy cells, and patients are often required to endure the sometimes severe side effects of large doses of multiple poisons for several months before the results can be measured. Inevitably some tumour cells will always be resistant to treatment, however aggressive the treatment may be. These cells may remain dormant for a considerable time before starting back into active growth.

This doesn't mean that all chemotherapies are ultimately a road to nowhere. Some do appear to work in the short term, although the results of studies in the long term, over 10 to 30, even 50, years have yet to be seen. Unfortunately, not all the doctors are willing to use the drugs on themselves. A much-quoted survey among a number of doctors in 1990 reported that the majority thought they would refuse chemotherapy if they were diagnosed with cancer (*The Cancer Chronicles*, December 1990).

Radiotherapy

Radiation is a word used to describe the emission of electro-magnetic waves as long-distance radio waves that are not considered to be damaging to body molecules, as atoms (non-ionising radiation) or as minute distance radio waves, the X-rays and gamma rays (ionising radiation). X-rays and gamma rays are capable of causing the formation of free radicals to kill both normal and mutant cells by rupturing their delicate outer membranes. This ionising radiation can damage any of your body molecules, either by killing the cells or by stimulating cell mutation that may also lead to cancer. However, the more rapidly dividing cells in an existent cancerous condition have been seen to be most susceptible to damage, which is why radiotherapy is recommended for treating some cancers.

Radiation can be delivered in several ways. These include: (a) high-voltage X-ray machines; (b) high-voltage linear accelerator machines; (c) surgically inserting radioactive isotopes as small, sealed units delivering very high, concentrated doses directly into a tumour or cancerous tissue; and (d) as unsealed radio-active sources usually administered in liquid form, either orally or as an injection. Unsealed sources are the most likely potential environmental contaminants, making a treated patient's bodily fluids highly radioactive during the first few days after treatment. Medical staff are issued with detailed instructions to avoid unnecessary exposure while caring for the patient, including careful handling and disposal of body waste, urine, faeces, etc. Hugs from visitors won't be allowed either.

The radiologist will carefully calculate the size and length of time of radiation doses with the intention of causing maximum damage to the cancer cells while inflicting minimum damage to surrounding healthy cells; the dose of radiation is measured in terms of absorbed energy. In terms of reference the *rad* (radiation absorbed dose) has been replaced by the *gray*, so that any reports you see may mention the dose in measurements of *gray* (100 rads = 100 centigray (cGy) = 1 gray).

Successful treatment very much depends on oxygen availablity in the tumour mass and the rate of cancer cell activity, as rapidly growing cellular tissue is more sensitive than tissue in which cells are dividing more slowly. X-ray and gamma ray therapies depend on the irradiated cells being well oxygenated, as the free radicals formed as a direct result of radiation exposure target the oxygen within the cells in order to bind and destroy cellular DNA. Plenty of oxygen can make cells as much as three times more sensitive to radiotherapy. Don't worry, only extremely large doses of between 30 and 100 *gray* will destroy your nervous system and kill you in a few days, something that is likely to happen only if you are directly exposed to the effects of an atom bomb or something similar.

You should be aware that not all cancers can be treated with radiotherapy. The sarcomas, melanomas and gastrointestinal tumours are generally considered to be the most radio-resistant, the least likely to respond to treatment. Lymphomas are among the most radio-sensitive and stand a greater chance of showing a successful result after treatment. Adenocarcinomas and squamous carcinomas have intermediate sensitivity, and respond according to type and condition.

Radium was the accepted radiation therapy during Rene's Cancer Clinic days in the 1930s. Some of the patients reported being given enormous doses of radiation, up to 36 hours of continual treatment at one time, and being 'burned to the bone' at the end of it. Radium has an almost unbelievable half-life of 1,620 years. This means that it takes 1,620 years for the amount of radioactivity emitted by radium to decline by half. It is hardly something you want to be around every day. Of course, you don't become 'radioactive' after treatment unless you are treated using one of the specialist unsealed radioactive sources as previously described, but can you wonder that handling radium on a regular basis killed its discoverer, Marie Curie?

Radium has now largely been replaced by Caesium-137 which has an environmentally and socially more acceptable half-life of 30 years. But 30 years is still 30 years, and radiation therapies are in regular use worldwide. Other 'radionuclides' include Iridium-192 with a half-life of 74 days, Iodine-125 with a half-life of 60 days, Iodine-131 with a half-life of eight days and Gold-198, with the most acceptable half-life of approximately 66 hours.

Questions to ask – in whatever order you like

- Is my tumour well supplied with oxygen?
- If it isn't, is it worth having the treatment?
- What will the treatment do to the rest of me in the long term?
- What are the chances of it working, and what quality of life can I expect during and after treatment?
- Am I being asked to take part in a drug trial, and why?
- If so, is this a completely new treatment, or has the drug been used for some time?
- What success rate has the drug showed with cancers like mine?
- Am I being offered the treatment to deal with a specific cancer, or am I being treated 'just in case'?
- Could you put me in contact with anyone else who has had the treatment?
- Doctor, do you know exactly what this treatment will do to me, and would you take it yourself?

At the end of the day, if a surgeon or an oncologist tells you there is nothing he can do for you, thank him for his honesty and his time and do not despair. He has just done you the great favour of sparing you pointless and vitally weakening treatment and given you back your time to work on your wellness. You are back on course to take charge of your own life with your cancer, with time to make room for the miracle.

What can I do?

There's a lot you can do. There's a lot you must do to get well. Miracles don't just happen to everyone else but you. Miracles do happen, and not always because of the intervention of various beneficent spirits. Miracles need some working on together with some active co-operation from the person who happens to be in need of one. Just sitting back and waiting for the doctor to cure you won't work. Both the doctor and the miracle need your help.

A cancer diagnosis isn't just about a tumour in one particular part of your body. Active cancer cells in one of your vital organs can trigger a domino effect – the idea that one event, if allowed to happen, will inevitably lead to a succession of similar events – in this case more cancer establishing itself in other parts of your body if you don't take care of your general well-being from the day of diagnosis.

All cancers have a life cycle, beginning with the mutation of the first cell and ending with the death of the tumour or the decline of the cancerous condition. You don't have to die with the cancer. Feed a cancer and you give it the opportunity of living forever. Henrietta Lacks contracted cervical cancer in the early 1950s. In 1951 cells cut out of her cancer were the first to be successfully cultured in a dish in a laboratory, and they are still growing, almost half a century since Henrietta's death. The well-fed 'HeLa' cells have become essentially immortal and continue to grow so vigorously in culture that they have become 'lab weeds', appearing as contaminants in other experiments in culture.

Your cancer is mortal. You are going to starve your cancer to give it the best possible chance of dying without taking you, the host, with it.

Feeding cancer

You can be unknowingly feeding cancer by what you eat, what you drink, where you live and how you live. And it's not just physical. What goes on inside your head matters just as much. Fear can kill you as equally effectively as cancer. The stress resulting from a depressed and passive attitude, and/or being frightened and lacking self-belief has been observed to have a direct effect on the body when dealing with apparently 'terminal' illness. Dr Laurence Badgeley (in *Healing AIDS Naturally*, 1987) reports:

- The thymus shrinks.
- The white blood cells decrease.
- The T-8 suppressor cells increase.
- The adrenals increase steroid production.
- Depression increases.
- The appetite decreases.
- The sex drive decreases.
- A constant fear and worry condition increases.
- Cancers grow faster.

Starving cancer

If a doctor tells you no one has ever recovered from your particular type of cancer, tell him there is no reason why you can't be the first. Medical records are notoriously inadequate in that they do not account for those who give up on conventional treatment and choose to remain unmonitored – and survive. A fighting, aggressive attitude will buy you time either to be there for the miracle or to die on your own terms. You will need a large helping of determination plus accurate information and a willingness to make some fundamental changes in your diet and general lifestyle. You are going to 'eat alkaline' and realise that healthy living doesn't have to be boring.

Begin by finding a reliable source of excellent, organic Essiac, well within the sell-by date time printed on the packet.

Better still, buy the individual herbs and start mixing and making up the tea for yourself. Correctly prepared Essiac has a pH value of 5, and is thought to begin its work by making the blood slightly more acidic. As your blood becomes acidic, your tissues become more alkaline. The opposite is also true. You want alkaline tissues because cancer does not thrive in an alkaline atmosphere. As such, Essiac in capsule form and in 'ready to use' tea bags that only need hot water and soaking can never be worthy substitutes for the remedial values of the stronger, correctly made decoction. If your energy levels are low, persuade your family and friends to help you make the tea until you are well enough to take over. Of course, no single remedy will be a blanket 'cure' for everyone, and Essiac is no exception. But the overwhelming weight of evidence in its favour makes it well worth trying when it is well done and the diet and lifestyle are rebalanced accordingly.

Remember, cancer does not happen overnight, so don't expect an overnight cure. Something that takes 10, 20 or even 30 years to establish will take time and care and consideration before it will go away. Some tumours grow so slowly that a cancer can be growing for many years before it is large enough to produce enough symptoms to make a doctor decide to send you for testing. The 1939 Toronto Cancer Commission Hearing records shows that some successfully treated patients attended the Bracebridge Clinic as many as 70 times over a period of up to two and a half years before they got results. Others got results in a matter of weeks. As always, all cancers are individual, and then, as now, results depend upon the circumstances unique to each individual diagnosis.

Question the therapies

Start by asking a lot of questions about the necessity of whatever surgery, chemotherapy or radiotherapy you are being offered. You don't want to be treated with something that will not only reduce your quality of life during and immediately after treatment, but may provide ample opportunity for new and more aggressive mutant cells to evolve. Ask for an honest assessment of the expected outcome of any proposed treatment, and then take time to think about it. Discuss it with your family if you want to before finally choosing for yourself.

SURGERY
Be brave and look at your scans, and ask the doctor to show you exactly what bits of you he is proposing to cut out before you next meet in the operating theatre. Try to start taking Essiac well before your operating date to give the tea the chance to draw as many of the cancer cells back to the primary site as possible. We have had many accounts of people doing particularly well after surgery, and occasionally of surgeons finding the cancer encapsulated and capable of complete removal when the patient has been taking Essiac, sometimes only after four or six weeks.

'Everybody in my family seemed to be getting cancer all around me, and I thought it was a good thing just to take Essiac as a preventative. So I'd been taking it, I guess maybe a year or two years, before I was diagnosed with bowel cancer. When they operated the doctor said the cancer was contained in a little pocket of its own, it hadn't spread any place and it was definitely curable. I've had no trouble since, and that was more than two years ago.'

Mr J. Hillman, Ontario, 1997

CHEMOTHERAPY
This can have a devastating effect on your blood cell count. We have had reliable reports of some doctors actually telling their patients to get hold of a good supply of Essiac and take it to bring their blood count back up to an acceptable level before they undertake further chemotherapy. Essiac is generally well tolerated alongside the various chemotherapies, and seems to make a marked difference to the patient's quality of life and general well-being during treatment. Don't forget to ask for information about any new chemotherapies not yet widely available. Sometimes doctors are sitting on supplies of a new

drug that is already being successfully trialled elsewhere. If you don't ask, you don't receive. At the same time, you must remember that unknown drugs can be more life-threatening than the disease. Don't volunteer yourself on to a drug trial on the grounds that you have nothing to lose. You do have something to lose – life and quality of life, and the miracle.

RADIOTHERAPY

This is generally well tolerated when the patient is taking Essiac, and energy levels are usually very well maintained. Some patients from the Bracebridge Clinic who made a full recovery from their cancer had been treated with radium. Remember to ask how much damage to surrounding normal tissue and vital organs can be expected, and ask the doctor to tell you how much serious damage to the tumour he truly expects to see as a result from the treatment.

'. . . *this (Essiac) is an excellent blood cleanser and can help tremendously if someone is toxic either from chemotherapy or radiation.*'

Dr Jesse Stoff,
An Alternative Medicine Definitive Guide to Cancer, 1999

Rebuilding your immune system

This is the first line of attack because by the time cancer is diagnosed, it means that the immune system cell structure, comprised of the macrophages, B cells, T cells and natural killer (NK) cells, has already been sufficiently weakened to allow the cancer cells to divide and multiply. You need to start producing lots of B cells for antibodies and lots of T cell types to help, particularly the CTL cells, which appear to have evolved specifically to attack tumour cells.

'*The role of the immune system in tumor suppression is further supported by the fact that immunosuppressed patients are more prone to develop cancer. For example, organ transplant patients, whose immune system is suppressed to prevent organ*

*rejection, have a threefold higher risk of cancer than persons
who are not immunosuppressed.'*
Dr Grant Steen, A Conspiracy of Cells,
The Basic Science of Cancer, 1993

Cut out the chemicals

Your lifestyle could have been seriously undermining your
immune system for years, but don't stress yourself unnecessarily
by trying to change everything overnight. Decide which changes
you can most easily manage immediately and gradually include
a few more as you start feeling better.

- Stop smoking and avoid a smoking atmosphere – not easy
  if you have been a smoker for most of your life, but it
  definitely helps. It has been estimated that as many as 30 per
  cent of all known cancers are directly or indirectly caused by
  exposure to the carcinogens in the tar in tobacco smoke.
- Filter your drinking water and boil it before drinking when
  you can. We get so used to the taste of chemically conta-
  minated water that it can be quite a shock to taste the real
  stuff. Ideally have an on-line filtering system fitted to your
  main water supply. Bottled water is easy to buy, but you
  should be aware that some bottled water can contain high
  levels of nitrates and radioactivity.
- If you can, get into the habit of using only pure soaps for
  washing yourself and your clothes. Stop colouring your
  hair and try washing it just once a week with pure and
  simple shampoos. If you have long hair – and people with
  cancer do have long hair – use a touch of sweet almond oil
  to help condition and shine dry hair. As you detoxify your
  body, you will find your hair condition will improve.
- Do your best to avoid eating residual pesticides by eating
  organic vegetables, organically supplied eggs (maximum
  twice weekly) and white meat and fish products. Wash
  your organic vegetables carefully before use to remove any
  traces of mould and giardia contamination, and stop

spraying your house plants and your garden with pesticides and weed killer.

- Keep your fluids flowing to avoid a build-up of toxic waste in your body. Cut all added salt (sodium chloride) out of your life and become aware of how your kidneys, liver and lymphatic system function.

- Remember that coffee and alcohol stress the liver and lymphatic system, and cut consumption down to a minimum. Better still, cut them completely out of your life.

Think thymus

The thymus is a rather neglected little organ located directly behind your breastbone, just over half way up between your heart and where your collarbones meet at the base of the throat. The thymus is prominent in young children, gradually shrinking as they reach maturity, but it doesn't go away and it doesn't stop working. The immune system cannot function without a regular supply of T cells produced from a healthy thymus. If negative thinking has been shrinking and twisting your thymus into a little knot in your chest, now is the time to think positive and big! It helps just to be aware that your thymus exists and is prepared to work with you, if you will allow it.

Look after your lymphatic system

If you were to light up and measure your lymphatic system you would see that you have up to 25,000 miles of lymph-bearing vessels quite literally all over your body, connected to the lymph-filtering nodes concentrated in groups in your armpits, groin, neck and around the main blood vessels in your abdomen and bowels. The lymphatic system is necessary to maintain drainage of excess tissue fluids and prevent protein levels building up in your tissue spaces, so causing fluid retention. Inflammation can also cause fluid retention, and if your tissues are predominantly acidic, your lymphatic system will be under-powered, over-saturated and toxic.

Cancer cells seem to thrive in over-saturated, toxic tissue spaces, and tumours are notorious at retaining fluid. There is no need to give them another excuse to retain more. Lymph vessels flow through muscles, so regular exercise, no matter how slow, will serve to pump the lymph back into your blood stream. However badly you may be feeling, don't lie in bed or on the sofa all day. Get up and walk around. Have at least five minutes of fresh air in your lungs every day, whatever the weather. Buy an exercise bike, set it up by a window so that you can enjoy the view and 'cycle' for at least two minutes every day, even at snail's pace – anything to keep your fluids flowing.

If you decide to have a massage to help drain the lymph system, make sure your practitioner is completely aware of your condition. Preferably only go to a practitioner who has a well-established reputation for dealing successfully with cancer patients. A well-intentioned but ignorant masseur may inadvertently facilitate the passage of mutant cells into the blood stream, the last thing you need if you have cancer.

Be kind to your kidneys

The pair of red–brown, bean-shaped organs either side of your spine and just above your waist are primarily responsible for controlling and maintaining the fluid and chemical balance in your body by filtration and selective reabsorption processes. The kidneys filter all the blood in your body approximately 20 times an hour, sending excess fluid and the waste products contained in that fluid to your bladder to be excreted as urine. Most drugs are eliminated through your kidneys, which may be exposed to high levels of carcinogens being removed from your blood. Drinking plenty of good water and paying careful attention to your diet can only help these hard-working little organs. The more water you drink, the less concentrated the waste products in your urine and the more frequent its excretion.

Learn to love your liver

Your liver is the largest organ in your abdomen and your main organ of chemical detoxification. It keeps down your internal pollution levels by producing enzymes to filter and transform the blood waste products and the toxins ingested from food, water, air, drugs and medicines, including chemotherapy, that cannot be handled directly by your kidneys. The liver enzymes transform these waste products so that they can be dissolved in water and be excreted in your urine and through your bowels. Insufficient enzymes and lack of antioxidants in the diet cause toxins to build up in the liver.

The liver is a delicate organ and not easy to operate on surgically as it has a complicated blood supply, but it does have a remarkable capacity for regenerating itself. Up to 80 per cent of the liver can be removed, and within a few weeks under favourable conditions it will have regrown sufficient tissue to compensate for the loss. Unlike most of the body organs, the liver is served by two major blood vessels: the hepatic artery carries approximately 25 per cent of all the nutrient and oxygen-rich blood from the heart to the liver; and the hepatic portal vein brings nutrients absorbed in the intestines directly to the liver. It supplies approximately 70 per cent of the total blood flow to the liver, collecting blood from capillaries in the spleen and the walls of the intestines, and draining both the small and large bowel. This direct link between the bowel and liver accounts for advanced colorectal cancers tending to metastasise to the liver. This direct link also serves to transport helpful substances from the intestines and the bowels to the liver.

Essiac has been found to be particularly effective in treating the liver. Dr Jesse Stoff, MD, writing in *An Alternative Medicine Guide to Cancer* (1999), believes that Essiac 'has an affinity for the liver and does not stress the kidneys'.

Care for your colon

Also known as your large intestine, the colon's main job is to conserve water absorbed from the contents of the bowel and

to promote the growth of healthy bacteria to synthesise vitamins. A high intake of dietary fibre increases the water content
of the bowel, speeding up and diluting any dietary carcinogens
through the bowel and cutting the risk of constipation. If you
have cancer, you don't need to be constipated. No one thrives
around blocked drains, and many of the conventional cancer
drugs and painkillers (particularly codeine and morphine) are
notorious for blocking the drains. Introduce a variety of beans,
whole grains and fresh fruit and vegetables into your diet rather
than just bran, which does not have much food value. Pulp the
foods in a kitchen processor if you have problems chewing.
Another option is to soak one teaspoonful of Slippery elm
powder in a glass of fruit juice for half an hour and drink it
before your main meal as a useful addition to your daily dose
of Essiac.

A qualified practitioner who is highly experienced in dealing
with people who have cancer can advise you on the various
colon-cleansing therapies if you feel you would benefit from
the treatment.

Understanding your drugs

It helps to know how drugs are administered and why, especially if you are sent home from the hospital with a bag full of
pills and potions and told to 'get on with it' yourself. The
unspoken rule that says we must read the fine print on
medication packs is rarely followed. We just open the bottle or
the carton, check out the least complicated part of the label to
find out how much and many times, and leave it at that. But in
accepting responsibility for using a drug, we should accept
some responsibility for how we choose or choose not to use
that drug.

ORAL THERAPIES – TABLETS, CAPSULES, LOZENGES
Tablets range from plain, white uncoated types to a complex
variety suited to particularly specific therapeutic assimilation.
If a drug is known to be a gastric irritant (likely to cause

stomach bleeding or gastric ulcers), it may be covered in a special coating enabling it to by-pass your gastric acids to be released into the small bowel. *Sustained release tablets* are designed to control the rate of release as the drug passes through the alimentary tract. *Capsules* usually contain drugs that are either difficult to make into conventional tablets or taste too nasty to be easily swallowed. If you are at home and responsible for your own drugs, you should be aware that unscored or coated tablets and sustained release tablets should not be broken or crushed, and capsules are better left intact. *Lozenges* are meant to be palatable enough to suck and are generally used for treating the mouth and throat. *Mixtures* are usually drugs suspended in flavoured solutions that need to be shaken before use to ensure the correct amount of the drug is included in each dose.

RECTAL THERAPIES – ENEMAS AND SUPPOSITORIES
Enemas are prepared solutions designed to be administered into the rectum either as laxatives or for localised therapeutic reasons. Sometimes enemas are used for diagnostic purposes. *Suppositories* are drug-impregnated, solid wax pellets designed to slip easily into the rectum before melting and releasing the drug into the bowel. Traditionally suppositories are used as laxatives, but they are increasingly used to administer many different sorts of drugs as they can be a useful alternative to drug administration by injection and are sometimes equally as effective.

VAGINAL THERAPIES – PESSARIES AND DOUCHES
Pessaries are drug-impregnated solid pellets designed to be inserted into the vagina, melting to release the appropriate drug for localised therapy. *Douches* are drugs diluted in solution to be administered directly into the vagina for localised therapeutic use.

TOPICAL THERAPIES – CREAMS AND OINTMENTS
Drugs to be applied directly to the skin are usually prepared in creams or ointments. *Creams* contain a high water content and

are rapidly absorbed into the skin. *Ointments* contain more oil and are absorbed more slowly, leaving a greasy residue on the surface of the skin.

INJECTABLE THERAPIES

Finally, a brief look at how and why injections are given. We are a needle-tolerant society, passively prepared to allow our bodies to be pricked and punctured in order to be 'cured'. Injections might hurt more than most therapies, but we tolerate them because we think they will do the job faster and more effectively. We never ask why. From early infancy we are conditioned to offer our arms and legs (and sometimes other parts of us) for injection with a sterile solution containing an active ingredient/ingredients, using a sterilised syringe and needle (selected according to how much we weigh, how much of us is muscle and how much of us is fat), as well as what sort of drug is scheduled to be stuck directly into us, using one of seven different routes:

- *Intra-arterial,* or directly into an artery. A rare and hazardous procedure sometimes performed to deliver a high drug concentration into a tumour mass.
- *Intra-articular,* or directly into a joint, which can be a painful treatment for acute, local inflammation.
- *Intrathecal,* or as used for administering local anasthetics, antibiotics, X-ray and chemotherapies into the cerebral spinal fluid.
- *Intravenous,* or directly into a vein, as in the administration of many chemotherapies.
- *Intradermal,* or into the upper skin layers, usually on the forearms where the layers are thin and where there is minimum hair. This method is mostly used for diagnostic testing as in the Mantoux skin test for tuberculosis.
- *Subcutaneous,* or injected beneath the skin into the fatty layers and connective tissue so that the drugs are absorbed slowly through the capillary network. The upper arm is usually the least painful site as there are fewer large blood vessels.

● *Intramuscular*, or direct into a large muscle mass. Drugs administered by this route can be rapidly absorbed and can produce blood levels similar to administration by intravenous method. Rene Caisse favoured administering the Sheep sorrel solution by intramuscular injection as near to the site of the tumour as possible.

Chapter Four

Diet – It Matters What You Eat

*T*here is at least a 15 per cent chance that what you have been eating has contributed to the establishment of your cancer. Unless you are prepared to make some changes to your regular diet, you may be continuing to unwittingly provide generous hospitality to an unwanted guest.

As far as we know, Rene did not offer any particular dietary advice to her patients during the days of the Bracebridge Clinic. They were given their weekly dose of Essiac and/or a Sheep sorrel injection, regardless of when or what they had last eaten. In spite of the growing pollution threat in the industrial areas in upstate, western New York, two hundred miles south of Bracebridge and from the nickel mine in Sudbury one hundred miles west, Rene's patients were not subject to the chemical cocktail that we routinely consume in our food today.

No matter who we are, a cancer diagnosis is always a shock. At such a time, we see the inevitable change in our lives as an invasion, a disempowerment. The last thing we want to do is to radically change our diet, the one area in our lives where we do have some control. Favourite food is comfort food. It is often easier to refuse to eat well than to refuse chemotherapy. Mali's husband Greg, who had spent most of his active adult life advocating complementary therapies and whole food diets, looked at the bewildering array of recommended diets and 'cures' he was offered when the brain tumour was diagnosed and refused them all on the grounds that 'too much of a good thing was no good at all'. His reaction was typical of someone recently diagnosed, very seriously ill and needing all his available mental, emotional and physical energy just to stay alive.

If Essiac is going to have maximum chance to do its job in our polluted, twenty-first century world, we must take a serious look at what we are feeding our bodies and maybe feeding the cancer as well. Most of the world's cancer incidence is concentrated within the sphere of the industrialised, so-called 'progressive' nations, and cancer is the price we appear to be paying for our collective greed. There are claims ranging from 15 to 60 per cent that of all cancers can be attributed to being diet-induced and diet-sustained. However, *there is no single remedial diet that is best for everyone.* Cultural environment, genetic make-up, even blood type can determine whether you are a meat needer or a vegetarian, and major dietary changes should be achieved over a period of time – obviously not a long period but sufficient to be accomplished with grace and respect for the person needing to make these fundamental changes. Someone who has existed primarily on burgers and chips cannot be expected to turn vegan overnight, and inflicting a grossly and previously unnatural diet on anyone as a result of a cancer diagnosis can only exacerbate the stress quota, something you don't need at any time and especially when you are fighting cancer.

Unfortunately, some of the specialist dietary therapies and information on these therapies are doubly confusing in that they appear to offer conflicting advice. They are also time-consuming and sometimes very expensive to maintain. If you are ill and living alone, spending hours juicing and stretching your reduced earnings to afford a complicated regime of dietary supplements is not always a viable option.

However, there is a 'golden thread' to be found at the heart of all confusion. Look after yourself by listening to what your body tells you it needs while observing a simple, sensible structure of preference. Your priorities must be: first, to maintain good energy and immune system levels; second, to achieve a reasonable amount of daily exercise to maintain muscle tone and structure; and third, to avoid unnecessary build-up of excess bodily fluids. Over-saturated and deoxy-genated tissue spaces put the immune system under stress and are more accommodating of toxic substances that they would not normally absorb.

Foods to avoid

FRIED FOOD, HEAVY STARCHES AND HIGH-PROTEIN FOOD

High-protein diets deplete the body's vitamin and mineral reserves and build up a large amount of toxic waste in vital organs and between the cells. Both high- and exceptionally low-protein diets can cause fluid retention and, over time, high-fat diets slowly starve the tissues of oxygen. Animal and culture experiments have indicated that fat can act as a cancer promotor.

SALT, AS IN SODIUM CHLORIDE AND ADDITIVES SUCH AS MONOSODIUM GLUTAMATE (MSG)

Excessive salt has a corrosive effect on the cells in the stomach lining, and a direct link between eating salty food and stomach cancer has been observed in different studies of the eating habits of different cultures around the world. Too much salt encourages fluid retention and possibly high blood pressure. Most processed foods contain added salt, MSG or both. You may think that you don't eat a lot of salt because you don't have a salt pot on the table, but you would be very surprised how eating processed foods raises the level of your daily sodium chloride consumption.

You need sodium, as naturally occurring in the food you eat, and potassium, working closely with magnesium in the body to balance your body fluids within the cells and between the cells and to control how much water should be excreted by your kidneys. When the balance is disrupted, the cells can either rupture from the entry of too much water or collapse if they don't get enough. Diuretic drugs are not the answer to fluid retention as they inhibit the body's reabsorption of vital minerals.

SUGARS

Eating sugar depresses your immune system and invites your cancer cells to a feast for up to five hours each time after you have eaten your favourite sweets, desserts, confectionery, chocolate, carbonated drinks and beverages, fruit squash, molasses, syrups, honey and jam. And don't even consider using artificial sweeteners instead.

GM FOODSTUFFS

All genetically modified foodstuffs represent an unknown quantity and should be avoided until time and research prove their worth. Unfortunately, this must include soya products. The May 2000 issue of *New Internationalist* reports that '75% of all herbicides used in the US are sprayed on corn and soya beans. The soyabean has been at the centre of the debate on genetically modified (GM) food. Soyabeans are found in 60% of our processed food from margarine to tofu.' Soya contains cancer-preventing isoflavones, but it has meaningful levels of natural phyto-oestrogens and contains phytates, which can prevent essential minerals such as calcium, iron, magnesium, iron and zinc being absorbed in the intestinal tract.

YEAST

Cut down on all yeast products and alcoholic drinks. Avoid live baker's yeast as live yeast cells deplete the body of the B vitamins and other nutrients. Bread contains salt, sugar and yeast, and consumption should ideally be avoided or limited to two slices each day.

RED MEATS

Avoid beef, lamb and pork products to prevent excessive toxicity in the colon and to help prevent a build-up of acidity within the tissues. In 1994, P. Toniolo *et al.* reported 'a causal relationship between red meat consumption and cancer', as supported by several comprehensive studies conducted in the USA.

SYNTHETIC FATS AND MARGARINES

Animal fats are most likely to contain many pesticide residues, and there is very little goodness left in the synthetic butter and margarine substitutes after they have undergone their heating, blending, bleaching, colouring and salting process. High-fat diets increase the possibility of your body producing its own damaging, oxygen-free radicals without the assistance of radiation and chemotherapy. Put away the deep fryer, develop a taste for cold-pressed Italian olive oil drizzled over your salads (because it is the best) and eat unsalted, preferably organic butter occasionally for treats. Dr Johanna Budwig recommends mixing flax seed oil with organic cottage cheese (add lemon peel zest for a delicious breakfast or desert) in order to make the unsaturated vegetable oil water soluble and easily assimilated as a remedy for a variety of serious medical conditions, including cancer.

STOP USING YOUR MICROWAVE

Originally developed during the World War II years, there have been so many conflicting reports on use of microwave ovens that utilise a power input of over one thousand watts to cook, defrost and reheat food. The resulting destruction and deformation of food molecules produces new, 'radiolytic' compounds, which are unknown in nature. It has been suggested that ingestion of microwaved foods causes a higher percentage of cancerous cells in human blood (W. Kopp, *J. Nat. Sci.* 1, 1998, 42–3). Dr Hans-Ulrich Hertel, a Swiss food scientist, is reported. as having discovered as far back as 1989 that 'any food that has been cooked or defrosted in a microwave oven can cause changes in the blood indicative of a developing pathological process that is also found in cancer'. Along with seven others, Dr Hertel took part in an eight-week extensive research programme that showed significant changes in the blood of those who had eaten microwaved food. The results of the study indicated blood levels symptomatic of a tendency towards anaemia, which became more pronounced and statistically significant during the fourth to eighth week of the programme.

Microwave ovens have become part of life, and reports such as these can be dismissed as scare-mongering when compared to the ease and time-saving aspects of the equipment – except for a story Greg told Mali before he died. Greg had spent seven years of his interesting and highly varied life as the abbot of a monastery in southern England. Many people from many different walks of life visited the monastery, including one American who was a scientist and claimed to be related to one of the first people to develop a commercially viable microwave oven in the USA. This man had carried out a study on the effect of microwaving food at his relative's request. As a direct result of his conclusions, his family decided to revert to conventional and traditional cooking methods. Greg remained sufficiently shocked and impressed by the man's story to make Mali promise never to use a microwave oven during her lifetime.

If you're fighting cancer, why risk adding to your problems? Store the microwave and get back into the habit of preparing food using traditional methods, like steaming and oven baking your food and including plenty of vegetables. Try to eat your fruit raw to retain the pectin content, which is vital in promoting the alkaline properties of the digested food.

Foods to eat

DRINK PLENTY OF WELL-FILTERED WATER

Your body is made up of 50 to 60 per cent water, and uses a complex system of hormones and prostaglandins to keep the fluid volume at a constant level. You need water to transport vital substances to where they are needed in your body, to transport waste products and to regulate your body temperature. Healthy kidneys need plenty of water to flush out toxins, at least three litres a day, mostly as plain water and in soups, fresh fruit juices (diluted up to 50 per cent with water), herb tea or green tea, milk alternatives such as rice milk or oat milk and, if you have a juicer, from your own fresh organic juices such as carrot, apple, grape, beet, orange and lemon juice.

Get into the habit of drinking a cup full of warm water as soon as you get up, before you eat or take any medication. The days of nothing but strong black coffee until lunchtime are over.

A VARIED DIET

You are aiming for a balanced, low-sodium, higher potassium/ magnesium diet that is moderate but not deficient in protein and contains sufficient fat as in the essential fatty acids (GLA) and in olive oil. Varying the diet helps to maintain your interest in food and avoids possible allergic reactions owing to repetitively eating the same foods. People Against Cancer (USA) suggest a high alkaline diet of 70 per cent vegetables, 10 per cent fruit, 10 per cent animal produce and 10 per cent grains.

Help your pancreas to produce its cancer-fighting enzymes by starting every meal with raw food if possible. Juice it if you have problems digesting it, and don't just stick at three meals a day. Graze on fresh fruit and nuts between meals to maintain energy levels. If you're hungry, eat. But remember to wash, scrub and peel your food, even organic food if you are not sure of the origin, to help reduce possible chemical residues.

ORGANIC FOODS

Do your best to eat organically grown foods. They are higher in potassium and lower in sodium than their artificially grown counterparts. Yes, we know organic foods tend to be more expensive, but have you ever wondered why all the cheaper vegetables laid out on the display shelves in the supermarket look so uniformly perfect?

For example: you owe it to yourself never to eat a non-organic banana because standard banana crops are routinely sprayed:

- eight to 12 times every year with herbicides, including glysophate, a suspected carcinogen;
- up to 40 times a year with fungicides, including manco-zebare, a suspected carcinogen;
- between two and four times a year with nematicides, which are extremely dangerous to people as well as to nematode worms;
- insecticides, impregnated into plastic bags and tags around the banana bunches;

- dipped in tisabendazol and aluminium sulphate as disinfectants after they are harvested.

And, of course, fertilizers are regularly applied to the fields throughout the year.

The people who harvest these bananas don't eat them and the bugs don't eat them. Neither should you.

LIFE WITHOUT COW'S MILK PRODUCTS

It is necessary to avoid IGF1, the only growth factor common to two mammals – cows and humans. IGF1 stimulates both normal and cancer cells into growth, and the growth factors are very different between cows and human beings. There is a huge difference in the growth and maturity of a one-year-old human baby and a yearling calf, and you don't need cow's milk telling your cancer cells to mature perhaps ten times faster than they might do. But don't panic about losing out on calcium because you've stopped drinking milk. Dairy produce can actually accelerate the rate at which the body loses calcium, and low levels of magnesium in the diet and coffee have been linked to osteoporosis. Coffee has the potential quite literally to dissolve away your bones. Yes, people drink a lot of strong coffee in the Mediterranean countries, but they are also drinking some of the 'hardest' water in the world, up to 30 per cent calcification in some parts.

On the other hand, whole grains, pulses, vegetables, nuts, eggs, kelp, spirulina and oatmeal provide meaningful amounts of calcium, which needs vitamin D and magnesium to ensure adequate absorption (this does not include eating a lot of bran, which can overly irritate your colon and prevent adequate absorption of calcium). Buying and consuming a moderate amount of organically produced goat's and sheep's milk products may provide a viable alternative to a life without cow's milk. There are also rice and oat milk alternatives to consider. It's just a question of re-educating and reconditioning your palate.

RED, GREEN AND YELLOW VEGETABLES
Eat all the red, orange, yellow and dark green fruit and vegetables you can manage, for the carotenes and flavanoids, vitamin C and vitamin E. These naturally occurring antioxidant foods protect the cells and minimise damage from free radicals.

A QUESTION OF PROTEIN
An average-sized man needs two ounces of protein a day. An average-sized woman needs one and a half ounces. High-protein diets stress the kidneys and the pancreas, but the liver depends on a continuing supply of protein to produce sufficient enzymes to process toxic waste. A healthy liver contains twice as much potassium as sodium, and an adequate supply of antioxidants in the diet will help to avoid toxic build-up in the liver. If the calorie intake falls, the protein intake must be maintained alongside a diet rich in whole grains, beans, pulses, fresh organic fruit and leaf and root vegetables to avoid liver over-detoxification. Several plant proteins should be combined, such as brown rice with lentils.

Shopping list

'*Red, yellow and green*' *fruit and vegetables*: broccoli, brussels sprouts, cabbage, cauliflower, kohlrabi, mustard, radishes and turnips, carrots, beets, spinach, cantaloup, papaya, peaches, asparagus, parsley, spinach, watercress, spring greens, sweet potatoes, pumpkin, endives, tomatoes, apricots, black grapes, black cherries, fresh apples, pears, raisins, prunes, wheatgrass and organic bananas.

Broccoli, cabbage and cauliflower stimulate the liver's biotransformation work. Beetroot, radishes and watercress stimulate the gall bladder to encourage the liver to drain itself into the intestines.

Natural sodium foods: organic kelp powder, fresh, deep sea fish, organically produced eggs, wheatgerm, celery and fresh 'red, yellow and green' fruit and vegetables.

Potassium foods: alfalfa, tomatoes, avocado pears, raisins, fresh 'red, yellow and green' fruit and vegetables, nuts (including cashew nuts), brown rice, spirulina and yams.

Magnesium foods: oats and oatmeal, which are also rich in B vitamins and dietary fibre, sesame seeds, almonds, alfalfa, whole grains, fresh 'red, yellow and green' fruit and vegetables, avocado pears and spirulina.

Zinc foods: carrots, beets, broccoli, cress, peas, beans, green vegetables, apples, deep sea fish, eggs, lentils, seeds, kelp, sprouted wheat and wheatgerm.

Selenium foods: organic grains (non-organic grains are often selenium-deficient), oats and cereals, fish, broccoli, cabbage, garlic, onions, radishes, sesame oil.

Raw foods are particularly alkaline and help the pancreas produce cancer-fighting enzymes. Juices and all raw fruits should always be eaten separately, at least two hours after eating other foods to facilitate maximum digestion and absorption levels

Raw juices place minimum strain on the digestive system and are absorbed into the blood stream almost as soon as they reach the stomach and small intestine.

Spirulina is the richest source of beta-carotene currently available and contains potassium, magnesium and iron in its molecular form.

Brown rice has 15 times the mineral content of white rice.

Wheatgerm is a good source of protein and vitamins as well as vitamin E.

Seaweed should be eaten at least twice a week as dried flakes scattered into salad.

Garlic lowers blood cholesterol levels, has antibiotic, anti-oxidant and anti-tumour properties and helps to flush harmful metals from the body. It also protects the liver from damage by synthetic drugs and chemical pollution. It is better raw than cooked, at least one clove daily. (Racehorses on garlic routinely return the best blood test results.)

Parsley is a natural deodoriser, rich in vitamin E and stimulates the kidneys.

Organic turmeric, the healing herb from India, has anti-bacterial qualities and contains curcumin, which has been shown to have anti-cancer activity as well as a protective effect on liver cells.

Organic kelp is an excellent source of vitamins and minerals, and is good for maintaining thyroid action, protects from the effects of radiation and helps to soften stools. Sprinkle the powder on salads.

Organic wholemeal flour has higher dietary fibre, phytic acid, protein and lipid content than white flour. Non-organic wholemeal flour may contain higher amounts of pesticides, mycotoxins and aerial contaminants because the outer husks of the wheat have not been removed during the milling process. So use organic unbleached flour for baking. Having cancer does not mean you are about to enter a culinary 'gulag' – you can still improvise with terribly healthy, minimum-sugar cake, scone and pancake recipes, and Christmas comes but once a year, which you can still enjoy with some degree of wisdom and moderation.

Supplements

Your body assimilates vitamins and minerals more directly from food sources than from pills and capsules. However, some supplements can help without necessarily breaking the bank.

● Vitamin A is best assimilated directly from the carotenoids in your food.

- Vitamin B complex, through diet, kelp and spirulina supplements.
- Vitamin B6 – cancer patients are often found to be deficient in vitamin B6. Take up to 100 mg daily.
- Vitamin C, up to 2 mg daily.
- Vitamin D, through diet, fish liver oils and sunlight.
- Vitamin E, 400 ius daily.
- Selenium, up to 200 mcg daily. Rene Caisse's Sheep sorrel was harvested from the selenium-rich soil around Bracebridge. We recommend anyone taking Essiac today to add selenium capsules to their shopping list.

Why green tea?

Green tea contains larger amounts of vitamins than black tea, including twice as much vitamin C. It also contains more than twice the catechins of black tea. Tea catechins have high vitamin P activity, and in 1987 epigallocatechin gallate (EGCG) was isolated as being the key protective ingredient in green tea. As an antioxidant, EGCG amounts to more than 50 per cent of total green tea polyphenols, which have been shown to 'inhibit viral replication at low levels, low enough to avoid destroying normal cells', possibly acting against free radicals to protect against tumour development. It may also prevent the activation of certain carcinogens so that free radicals never form. In one experiment,

'Mice that drank green tea instead of plain water for ten days before and during exposure to ultraviolet light proved less susceptible to skin damage.'

Z.Y. Wang *et al., Carcinogens* 12, 8, 1991, 1527–30

Green tea consumption has been monitored in studies in Japan, which have shown links between areas of higher, habitual tea consumption and a markedly lower incidence of stomach cancer in comparison with areas where tea consumption is less. Hirota Fujiki, a chemist at the National Cancer Centre Research Institute in Tokyo, goes so far as to say:

'This green tea cannot prevent every cancer, but it is the cheapest and most practical method of cancer prevention available to the general public.'

Green tea may be good for:

● its therapeutic effect on infectious diseases, including dysentery;
● treating rheumatism, with a favourable effect on both general condition and capillary resistance;
● its 'favourable regulatory effect on every vital component of human metabolism';
● enhancing immunity and destroying bacteria through the action of polyphenols, with strong anti-viral and antioxidant effects;
● reducing instances of pancreatic and stomach cancers;
● it 'may reduce the risk of some forms of human cancer induced by both physical and chemical environmental carcinogens', according to Z.Y. Wang *et al.*

Be inventive with your food, budget carefully and don't feel guilty if you cannot afford an army of vitamin and mineral supplements. Avoid selling techniques that pressurise you into unlimited spending 'if you value your health', and don't become so fanatical about your diet that you stop enjoying the occasional invitation out to eat whatever is on the menu. You have to eat in order to stay alive, so eat and eat wisely – and don't forget to have fun.

Chapter Five

Your Essiac Questions Answered

Preparation

Why are the exact proportions so important when making up Essiac?
The exact proportions are important for Essiac's synergistic effect to achieve full potency and because the remedy has been demonstrated to be well tolerated at these proportions using Rene Caisse's recommended dosage levels.

For those who cannot afford to purchase expensive stainless steel equipment, which is the most important item for someone on a limited income?
The pot is the most important item and will preferably be made of enamel, ceramic, heat-resistant glass or stainless steel in that order, the size depending on how much Essiac you plan to make at one time. The pot must have a well-fitting lid. Do not use teflon-coated cookware when preparing the tea.

Does a dark brown brew indicate that older, less potent herbs have been used to make the tea?
No. At the same time, Essiac is not supposed to be dark brown. The quality and correctness of herbs supplied should be questioned, remembering that an overly large proportion of Burdock could turn the decoction dark brown. The large bottle in the photograph on the front cover contains essiac made up

to the accepted colour. Very occasionally it may be greenish in colour.

What quantity of Burdock seeds do you recommend using in addition to the prepared four herbs?
If you can obtain organic seeds, add literally a pinch of Burdock seeds per half-ounce of the dry herbal mix.

Why did Rene insist on diluting Essiac?
Essiac is a herbal decoction. By its very nature, any herbal decoction is concentrated and strong. Bearing in mind that individual people will have differing tolerance levels to any form of concentrated decoction, Rene always advised diluting Essiac in hot water to make a pleasant and soothing drink before going to bed.

Cancer rates in Europe and USA/Canada are higher in some areas than others through many factors, possibly including soil and water contamination. Should this be taken into consideration when deciding to grow your own Sheep sorrel?
Of course it must. But sometimes it is better to know where the herb has come from and how it has been harvested and stored rather than to accept a non-organic product of dubious viability that just happens to be the only product the store has available at the time.

Considering that herbalists say that soft tissue herbs should neither be boiled nor powdered in order to retain potency, and most modern-day Native American medicine men prefer to use coarsely cut herbs, how did Rene Caisse justify powdering and boiling the Sheep sorrel when preparing Essiac? Why was she so adamant that the herb should be powdered?
The original Native American medicine man made the first eight-herb recipe exclusively for the benefit of a single woman patient. Rene Caisse took the recipe and developed it into Essiac, working with and developing each herb through a process of trial and elimination. She was not a herbalist. She

was a nurse and trained in the early twentieth century to work with doctors who still relied on using a percentage of herbal preparations when treating their patients. She did not work like a herbalist or think like a herbalist, yet the records from the Toronto Government Hearings of 1939 indicate positive results over a broad spectrum of cancers far exceeding anything recorded by herbalists before or since. In her letters to Dr Stock at MSKCC, she insisted that the herb was prepared by being coarsely powdered and boiled in decoction for the injections, the use of which have undoubtedly produced the best Essiac results to date. So far our 'active' research has shown that the decoction of the dried and powdered herb appears to be more potent than preparations using the fresh leaves, as though the limited oxidisation process involved during the drying and storing procedures adds to the efficacy of the herb in therapy.

However, there is a difference between wet heat and dry heat, in this case a little bit like the difference between burning toast and boiling potatoes. Unless it is carefully monitored, the grinding process can subject the herb to an almost scorching heat and over-oxidisation, which may destroy the constituent quality of the herb, especially if it is going to be stored for any length of time.

What proportions of herbs to water should a person use to ensure good preservation in storage if they are only going to take 30 ml a day for 10 days and then reduce the dose to 15 ml?
Mixing half an ounce in weight of the dry herb mixture with one and a half litres of water will last one person taking 30 ml daily for just over a month. The decoction stores best in the fridge in smaller bottles holding 250–300 ml of the decoction.

I have been told that taking Essiac in tincture form is not as effective as the decoction. What can you say about this, please?
A student herbalist sent this letter to Sheila:

'I was talking to another person experienced in the use of Essiac, who told me that Essiac only works in the form of the decoction and that the tincture is not as effective. This makes

sense to me as I have only used the decoction myself, making it in the same way as Rene Caisse, but I know of other people who have been using the tincture. The decoction is boiled while the tincture is simply an alcoholic extract and is not heated at all. Obviously different medicinal substances have different physical properties, and I would guess that the medicinal properties in Essiac need to be boiled to bring them out and to allow the various ingredients from the four herbs to interact with each other *during the boiling and steeping processes, producing new substances not necessarily exclusive to any one of the original ingredients – the synergistic effect.'*

Blood

Does Essiac affect the blood by thinning it or thickening it?
It appears to have the capacity to do both, depending exactly on the nature of each individual case. Essiac's ability to reduce haemorrhage has been documented since Rene first began experimenting with the Essiac herbs. Equally we have had reports of people already on drugs to thin the blood and reduce clotting, having to reduce their daily dose because the original, higher dosage level had become no longer necessary.

Will I risk increasing the chance of having a stroke if I take Essiac?
The correct herbs taken at the recommended dosage levels to date have shown no propensity for increasing risk of stroke. We do know of people who have a long-term history of high blood pressure finding their blood pressure readings normalising while taking Essiac.

Dosage

What guidelines do you suggest for dosage? How long should I expect to take the tea, and when can I reduce the dose to the 15 ml maintenance levels?
Rene recommended the 30 ml daily dose for cancer. Depending on the exact nature and severity of your condition, you may

have to consider taking Essiac at this dosage level for a period of up to two years, with 'resting' intervals of perhaps one week off in every four in order to stimulate maximum efficacy of the tea.

Can higher Essiac doses actually do more harm than good, and why?
It is our experience that the body seems to resist Essiac at higher doses. Rene Caisse considered high doses a complete waste of the remedy and risked the possibility of stimulating over-detoxification crises.

When Rene was conducting her research with Essiac, world pollution levels were considerably lower and food sources were less liable to residual contamination. Does living in our polluted, stressful present-day world justify a higher daily preventative dose of the tea?
No, we don't believe it does. If anything, higher daily doses may add to the bodily stress factors when processing toxic waste material.

Diet and supplements

If Essiac users are supposed to drink more than the recommended daily requirement of 64–80 fluid ounces of water, would you specify exactly how much and when?
If you are taking Essiac, you are detoxifying to a greater or lesser degree, depending on your condition. It makes sense to drink as much pure water as you feel comfortable with during the day, and take your Essiac last thing at night before you go to sleep in order for it to do its work undisturbed while your body and mind are resting.

Estimating your daily liquid requirement is made easy using an accepted rule imported from the USA: Body weight in pounds divided by two = the number of fluid ounces of liquids required. Someone weighing 120 lb/54 kg would need 60 fl oz of liquids a day.

Why should other beverages not be substituted for plain water?
They can be, as long as plain water is drunk regularly every day and tea, coffee and alcohol are cut down to a minimum. Ideally up to 70 per cent of your diet can be made up of water-rich food as in fresh fruit and vegetables and/or their freshly squeezed juices. Eat a salad with every meal and snack separately on fruit instead of sweet bars and crisps. Don't drink fluids with meals as you will dilute your digestive juices and slow up the digestive process.

Why should Essiac users restrict their consumption of tea and coffee and alcohol?
Essiac users can drink as much green tea as they like, without milk and sugar (see pages 108–9). Black tea has some value but only if drunk without milk and sugar. A squeeze of lemon makes a refreshing addition. Coffee stresses the liver and the lymphatic system and should be avoided. Alcohol depletes the body of magnesium, vitamin B complex and vitamins C, D, E and K.

Did Rene Caisse give other advice besides taking the tea, such as the importance of diet, vitamins and minerals?
No, not as far as we know. Remember that she was primarily a product of the 1920s and 1930s, when vitamin and mineral supplements were largely unheard of and diet was generally unresearched.

Will vitamin and mineral supplements, other herbs or any other foods interfere with the efficacy of the tea, even if taken at other times of the day?
Not generally. Essiac is usually very well tolerated with other therapies as long as it is taken separately from them so that it has maximum chance of achieving its full potential effect. We must point out, however, that we do not advise mixing Essiac with Chinese herbal therapies because the contents of the latter are often only known to the therapist who is prescribing them. Some of the more potent Chinese herbs may set up an extremely toxic reaction when used in conjunction with Essiac.

Combination therapies

I have been using the Gerson therapy coffee enemas four times a day for the past two months. Can I use the Sheep sorrel solution as an enema at the same time?
No, we would definitely not advise the use of the two remedies together, and we do question the advisability of using coffee enemas at such levels for this length of time. According to James and Phyllis Balch (*Prescription for Nutritional Healing*), excessive use of coffee enemas over a period of time can cause anaemia in healthy people – and that's only using the enema once a day. Why should cancer patients be any the less at risk? If you wish to start using the Sheep sorrel solution, it would be best to stop using the coffee enemas completely and wait for at least two days before starting with the Sheep sorrel enemas. Use them as advised, 10 ml of the solution diluted in 20 ml water at blood heat once every three days. Lubricate the tip of the enema with the oil from a 200 iu capsule of vitamin E, which will have a healing effect on the tissue lining the anus and the colon.

Should I continue to take Essiac while I am having radiation therapy?
Yes. Many people have reported tolerating the side effects of radiation well both during and after treatment time. Applying undiluted sheep sorrel solution to the skin immediately prior to radiation treatment lessens the possibility of the skin breaking down at the point of entry of the ray.

Is there a more beneficial time to begin taking the tea, i.e. before or after chemo/radiotherapy?
Any time is beneficial but the sooner you start, the better chance you have of benefiting from the tea. Take it before, during and after treatment.

Would you please comment on the use of hydrazine sulphate, laetrile and Mistletoe–Isacador therapies used in combination with Essiac?
Hydrazine sulphate: easily available by mail order in capsule form, we have heard this cheaply produced, common industrial

by-product labelled as 'do-it-yourself' chemotherapy. Our first question concerning the use of hydrazine sulphate has to be: 'what about its long-term effects on the liver?'

Mali collected some interesting responses from people who had contacted Joseph Gold's Syracuse Clinic for advice on using the chemical. A lady with ovarian cancer was advised that she could take the treatment and that using Essiac in conjunction with hydrazine was fine. Another lady with lung cancer was also advised she could take the treatment, especially in combination with Essiac. When Mali called the clinic and asked about the effects of hydrazine sulphate in combination with Essiac on the liver, she was told 'very warmly' that Essiac was 'really good' to take under such circumstances. These reports suggest that Essiac might be useful in palliating any possibly adverse side effects of hydrazine sulphate on the liver. The only person who was immediately advised to consult her doctor before taking hydrazine sulphate was a lady who had liver cancer. The adviser did not mention using Essiac as a combination treatment.

We have had reports of people using hydrazine sulphate to relieve pain, to stimulate the appetite and to stabilise tumour growth levels. So far, those who have noticed reduction in tumour size or blood count levels while taking hydrazine have seen tumours start back into growth and CA125 levels for ovarian cancer rising during periods without taking the chemical.

Laetrile: the word 'laetrile' (laevo-rotatory nitriloside) was originally coined to patent a particular injectable preparation of amygdalin, found in apricots, peaches and bitter almond kernels. This injectable therapy was the only therapy that showed significant results with cancer. Sweet almond kernels do not contain amygdalin. In *Cancer Therapy*, Ralph Moss says: 'There can be no argument that when eaten to excess or taken orally, amygdalin can be dangerous . . . under enzymatic action, amygdalin breaks down into glucose, benzaldehyde and hydrogen cyanide.'

It is possible that taking as few as 12 raw apricot kernels at one time could be dangerous. We have no reports of any adverse effects when combining 'laetrile' (amygdalin) food substances with Essiac, presuming that the person is using the amygdalin in a safe and acceptable manner.

Mistletoe–Iscador: in Europe, a small percentage of cancer patients who are actively pursuing complementary cancer therapies are treating themselves using oral Essiac combined with courses of Iscador injections. Iscador is the most widely marketed mistletoe preparation, containing extracts of fermented European mistletoe (*Viscum album*) combined with minute, homeopathic doses of copper, mercury and silver. We have had no reports of any adverse reaction when combining these two therapies.

Can I use Essiac if I am following the Hulda Clark method?
People do. We have no personal experience of this, but those who have reported to us seem satisfied with however they have integrated the two in combination. We are having some interesting reports of people combining the Royal Raymond Rife electrotherapy treatments with Essiac. If you can find a doctor or practitioner who is experienced in using the equipment, this combination therapy is well worth considering.

Questions concerning contraindication

If some essiac derivatives have a potentially high iron accumulation level, should people with heart conditions, diabetes or liver disease use Essiac?
In 1926, Dr Banting (who pioneered the use of insulin for diabetes), having examined the notes from a diabetic/cancer patient Rene had successfully treated during the previous year, said that 'Essiac must actuate the pancreatic gland into normal functioning. Otherwise the patient would have had to take treatments for the rest of her life, just as she would have had to take insulin.'

We know of people with heart conditions and serious liver complaints who have suffered no ill effects and appear to have thrived using Essiac prepared in the correct proportions and used at the correct dosage levels.

Why shouldn't Essiac be taken during pregnancy and during lactation?
As always, caution must be exercised. However, Essiac was reported to have been administered to a 19-year-old pregnant woman suffering from a rare form of cancer of the jaw, 'rhabdomyosarcoma'. Considering the mother's condition and the chemotherapy she underwent, the odds against the baby's survival were estimated at 4,000 to one. As soon as the Essiac treatment began, the mother's condition improved sufficiently to successfully deliver a healthy baby girl. The mother died a month later. Her family gave full credit to Essiac for enabling her to recover sufficiently to bring the pregnancy to a successful conclusion.

Besides pregnant and lactating women, who should be recommended not to take Essiac?
In our experience, Essiac is widely tolerated for a variety of complaints. However, we do advise people with osteoarthritis never to use more that 15 ml/half a fluid ounce daily, to be taken during the day rather than last thing at night, and always to take combination fish oils as a supplement. People with rheumatoid arthritis seem to do particularly well when using this Essiac/fish oil supplement combination therapy.

Should I take Essiac if I have kidney cancer?
Yes, you can, as long as your Essiac is correctly prepared in the right proportions and you take the correct dose of one fluid ounce a day. We have had several reports of kidney cancers being successfully treated with Essiac.

Concerning oxalic acid, James Duke lists it as antiseptic, CNS-paralytic, homeostatic, irritant, pesticide and renotoxic. Would the oxalic acid content in the herbs make Essiac potentially toxic to existent or underlying kidney conditions?
Essiac does not consist purely of oxalic acid. Again, when the correct herbs are used at the correct dosage, we have found no reports of kidney damage, either past or present. Mali has been

taking Essiac almost continually as an experiment for over seven years, and her inborn weakness of the right kidney has shown no sign of deterioration.

In his *Advanced Treatise on Herbology* Dr Edward Shook states:

'Oxalic acid does not occur free in nature, but is found in combination with sodium, potassium, calcium, iron and manganese in the juices of many plants such as rhubarb, sorrel, oak bark, cinchona, yellow dock etc.'

Charlotte Erichsen-Brown, in *Use of Plants for the Last Five Hundred Years*, writes:

'By periodic examination of the leaves of ascorbic acid and oxalate rich plants of the Polygon and Rumex families, it was determined that during growth, the ascorbic acid and oxalic content increased or decreased in parallel. This was especially true of Polygonaceae whose high oxalate content, between 2500 mg and 3500 mg per hundred grams of fresh leaves, coincided with a high ascorbic acid or Vitamin C content.'

It has been said that too much of a good thing is no good at all. Would you please comment on a recently reported case of a gentleman who had been using Essiac continually for a considerable period of time? Taking the tea helped him at first but by not alternating with other treatments or stopping at regular intervals, it is alleged that the tea has damaged the lining to vital organs (kidney, stomach etc.).

We have never heard of any similar case, and we have found nothing in the archives to suggest such a possibility occurring. To answer we would have to question the source of the allegation and the condition of the patient, and also to question the quality of the tea and the dosage levels he was using.

Is there any form of cancer that Essiac appears to have little effect with?

Essiac's primary function appears to boost the immune system and stimulate feelings of well-being in whoever is using the tea, as well as possibly providing some general remedial value in treating cancerous conditions. Considering this, Essiac may have some beneficial effect on any cancer, both primary and metastatic, depending on the individual person.

Is it really so important that patients be monitored closely by a health professional while taking Essiac?

It is our experience that most health professionals excuse themselves from monitoring Essiac because they say they have had no formal training in the use of the remedy. The decision to take Essiac is one of personal choice, and valuable in that it reinforces the desire and self-belief in the individual to take responsibility for their own life with their illness. As such, the judgment of a well-qualified professional who can maintain an impartial viewpoint while monitoring the treatment would be extremely valuable for research purposes, as long as the individual's right to decide upon and consent to treatment is not hindered in any way.

Historical

If the Private Members Bill put before the Toronto Parliament in 1938 had been passed, would Essiac have been legally recognised as a cure for cancer in Canada?

No, it would not. The Act requested to 'authorise Rene Caisse to practise medicine in the Province of Ontario in the treatment of cancer and conditions therein'. No mention was made of the specific use of Essiac as a remedy for cancer because no parliament could sanction the use of a remedy or therapy without knowing exactly what it consisted of. Had the Act been passed, presumably anyone other than Rene who was dispensing Essiac to treat cancer may have been liable to prosecution at that time.

What were the exact figures for the 1937–38 petitions and how many were actually submitted?

There were a total of seven petitions signed on Rene's behalf as follows:

- 27 October 1926, eight doctors signed a petition to be presented to the National Health and Welfare Department in Ottawa.
- 9 August 1935, 2,700 people signed a petition to be presented to Queen's Park Parliament in Toronto.
- 10 July 1936, 4,100 people signed the Bracebridge petition, presented to Parliament in Toronto.
- 31 October 1936, a petition was signed by three doctors and four business representatives, two in Cobden, Ontario, one in Toronto and one in Bracebridge, totalling seven signatures in all, presented to Parliament in Toronto.
- 23 December 1936, nine physicians signed another petition on Rene's behalf.
- 15 March 1937, 17,000 people signed a petition, presented to the Parliament in Toronto.
- 22 February 1938, 28,000 people signed a final petition, presented to Parliament in Toronto, including approximately 300 patients and 40 doctors.

A total of 51,824 names appeared on petitions on Rene's behalf, but this figure does not allow for repetition. Some people signed all four petitions.

Chapter Six

Tea Stories

Tea stories past

An Essiac book would not be complete without another look into Rene's six surviving case books from the Bracebridge Clinic records. We have chosen a variety of testimonies to include as evidence for Essiac being used for goitre, stomach and leg ulcers. Two of the cancer patients were still alive in 1977 and were both more than happy to give Sheila an update on their condition.

CANCER OF THE LIP

Book One, Page 1
Mr Tony Baziuk, Age 36 years, Capreol, Ontario.

Physician: Dr McNeill, London, Ontario.
Diagnosis: cancer of the lip (and stomach ulcers).
Remarks: patient had radium treatments at London, Ontario. Patient's face was so disfigured it was unbearable to look at when he first came to the clinic. Had first 'Essiac' treatment, 19 September 1936, weight on that date 151 lb. After the first treatment, the growth on the lip entirely disappeared. After one month the patient came to the clinic for a second treatment. On his second visit, the face was normal and people did not know him. He improved rapidly and gained in weight.

Copy of an article in the Bracebridge Gazette *of 17 February 1938*

A GRATEFUL PATIENT OF MISS CAISSE

Mr Tony Baziuk, C.N.R. engine watchman at Capreol, called at the *Gazette* Office recently. He was in town to bring down a largely signed petition from Capreol on behalf of Miss Rene M. Caisse and to express his heartfelt thanks to her. Mr Baziuk tells the *Gazette* his experience as follows:

About a year ago he had cancer of the lower lip so badly he could see the swollen lip over the end of his nose and he had been compelled by his suffering to quit his railroad job and go on relief. A locomotive engineer happened to notice Mr Baziuk's lip and told him he should come to see 'that nurse in Bracebridge'. So Mr Baziuk managed to get to Bracebridge with the aid of friendly railroaders and went to Miss Caisse. He took five treatments and felt relief two hours after the very first treatment. One week later he was able to go back to work for the C.N.R. and has been on the job ever since. He took the last treatment in April 1937. He feels healthy now and says: 'I eat for one man and work for three and sleep like a little baby'. Such is the experience Mr Baziuk related to the Gazette one day last week and he certainly does not seem to have anything unusual now about his lower lip, except a small hollow at the right corner where he says the cancer was.

12 October 1938: patient very well, eats anything he wishes without distress. Has worked since taking the first 'Essiac' treatment, was unable to work previously to that. Lip looks perfectly normal.

At the bottom of the page in Rene's handwriting: 'Patient still living, 1960'.

Sheila went to visit Mr Baziuk in 1977:

'When I met Tony in 1977, he was in his 80th year (he was born 19 November 1898). A hole on the right side of his lower lip serves as a reminder of the cancer that grew there in 1936.

He recalled very clearly how his lip became so swollen after only one radium treatment that he could see it over the end of his nose. Pain kept him off work and he was unable to eat. With $1.00 in his pocket, he went to Toronto by train for a check-up. At the Union station, a friend told him about Rene Caisse in Bracebridge. He had no money left so he was given a free train ride and arrived at the clinic. He felt immediate relief after the first injection, and felt even better when Rene gave him $5 because she knew he was flat broke. Six months later he was back at work and could 'eat for one man, work for three (at 46 cents an hour) and sleep like a little baby'. A musician who can't read a note of music, Tony had built 16 harps and a violin, playing both instruments with remarkable ability.'

MULTIPLE TUMOURS, BREAST, UTERUS, STOMACH

Book One, Pages 10, 11, 12, 13
Mrs May Henderson, Age 41 years, 10, Chicora Drive, Toronto.

Physicians: Dr Diack and Dr Barclay, Women's College Street Hospital, Toronto; Dr J.A. McInnis, Timmins, Ontario.
Diagnosis: fibrous tumour in breast and side, also large uterine tumour – Dr McInnis considered it malignant.
Remarks: patient had goitre operation but no other operation or treatment. When patient came to Miss Caisse, she was run-down, weak, muddy-like colour of skin and having great loss at menstruation time with haemorrhaging. Weight was 115 lb. First treatment by 'Essiac', 10 April 1937.
24 April 1937: patient's weight 118 lb, looking and feeling better.
9 May 1937: patient had haemorrhage at menstruation time.
19 July 1937: patient feeling improved, is working every day.
October 1938: patient feeling very well and working every day, growths almost entirely disappeared. Has had no other treatment except 'Essiac'.

At the bottom of the page in Rene's handwriting: 'Patient still living 1960'.

Mrs Henderson confirmed her recovery in a letter to Rene Caisse in October 1938:

October 18 1938
Miss Rene Caisse, The Cancer Clinic,
Bracebridge, Ont.

My dear Miss Caisse:

I am giving herewith particulars of my long and rather bad health history. Am arranging them in order according to dates as it seems to me now that I try to set down the particulars that ever since I have grown up I have suffered growths in some part or other of my body. As a child I enjoyed splendid health and was really conscious of being unusually strong. I thoroughly enjoyed a real tussle with my two brothers, both near my own age and never remember any sickness to speak of until the first periods appeared.

1910 – At this time I was fourteen years of age and a goitre appeared in my throat. From that time on I was never very well.

1922 – At this time a condition appeared in my left breast which forced me to go to my doctor (Dr Isabella Woods). She told me she did not know what it was and to come back in a month's time. I was very frightened and went to see another doctor (Dr Charles B. Parker). He pronounced it 'chronic mastitis' and gave me medicine to take internally and to apply to the breast. It relieved the condition for a time. He also discovered the goitre in my throat and advised an operation. I consented and had it removed early in 1923.

1931 – The mastitis continued to give me trouble and by this time a 'cystic' mass had formed, and in the right breast a tumour as large as a hen's egg. In March of 1931 I went to five different doctors (Drs Parker, Shouldice, Sullivan, Robt Gaby, Robinson), all of whom agreed that there was nothing known to science that would clear up the condition. There was no alternative but to have both breasts removed. I simply could not face it.

1935 – At this time and for some years prior I had had a severe haemorrhage every month until again I was forced to go to a doctor. I went to the Women's College Hospital Clinic and was examined by Dr Helen Diack and her co-worker, Dr Barclay. I was quite surprised when they had me on the table for examination to see a lump as large as an ordinary sized grapefruit in my right side. They told me it was a fibroid tumour and would of course have to be removed at once. There was also a smaller, long-shaped growth in the left side close to the hip-bone. I asked Dr Diack particularly about this as I was quite sure it was a different type of growth to the other side. She turned her head away and merely said, 'Well of course, it will have to come out too.' Needless to say by this time I was really very sick.

1936 – Early in the year a friend told me of the wonderful work being done in the Cancer Clinic at Bracebridge. Without any diagnosis or other letter to yourself, Miss Caisse, I came in a hurry. You told me that you had to have a written diagnosis from a medical doctor, and that I would have to undergo an examination by a doctor who would be in the Clinic the following week. This I did and I have just lately (and by accident) found out that he considered my case too far gone altogether to respond to any treatment. He did not examine my breasts or he would have found a small but well-developed cancer at the top of the left breast. By this time it was all I could do to be up and around at all. I haemorrhaged so badly I thought I would die, and I spent more and more time on the Chesterfield or in bed, and could lay down and sleep at any time of the day. My colour was a muddy, yellow colour, hair thin and lifeless, and eyes – ordinarily blue – were grey and stony looking. I simply couldn't stand up for any length of time as the feeling of weight and the weakness of the whole of the front of my body was unbearable. I did not suffer much pain but occasionally a sharp, needle-like stab would go through me around the growths. A movement of the bowels was frequently very painful though not always. I have suffered from constipation all my life.

1937 – And now for the happy ending: The growths have almost entirely disappeared, I have gained ten pounds and I feel fine. I go to work every day in a very busy office, where the staff are unaware that there is a thing the matter with me. Hours are from 8.30 to 5.30 and I get pretty tired at times, especially when, as at the end of the month, I work an evening or two. Then on Sunday there is the long trip to Bracebridge and back. If only I could rest on Sundays I feel sure I would make even better progress. I am, however, deeply grateful for the treatments and feel that I can never repay in money what they are worth to me. You have given me back my life, Miss Caisse, but what means even more to me, I can confidently look forward to perfect health so I shall enjoy living.

I think I have made it clear from the foregoing how utterly futile operations would be in a case like mine. My earnest prayer every day is that this remedy may be made available to every one who needs it.

Yours very truly,
Signed (Mrs) May Henderson

Mrs Henderson had written to the Prime Minister on Rene's behalf in July 1937, and when Sheila met her in Toronto in 1976, she was 80 years old and still actively campaigning for official recognition for Rene and Essiac. They visited the Toronto Parliament Buildings together at Queen's Park to talk to Margaret Campbell in the Premier's Office in another attempt to lobby for support for Rene.

KIDNEY CANCER WITH DIVERTED COLITIS

Book Three, Page 6, Case 5
Mrs A.G. Cameron, Age 56, 15, Roblock Avenue, Toronto, Canada.

Physician: Dr S. Sommacal, Toronto, Ontario.
Diagnosis: cancer of left kidney, diverted colitis.
Normal weight: 120 lb.
Remarks: patient examined at Western Hospital, Toronto by eight or nine doctors, also examined at Lockwood Clinic,

Toronto. Patient had all kinds of X-rays, has no radium, no operations, in very nervous condition, diverted colitis.

A letter dated 2 April 1936 from the Lockwood Clinic verifies Mrs Cameron's condition:

'. . . *we were quite satisfied that she had a good sized growth or tumour of the left kidney, probably of a malignant nature and that the condition should be attended to with as little delay as possible, surgery being the only thing which would promise her a cure. A delay of six months in having this done would probably render the case too late for successful surgery, as metastases, that is spreading of the growth through the blood stream, would be very likely to occur in this time.'*

First 'Essiac' 7 June 1937.

17 August: 'patient reports having sloughed off a piece of real tissue and has had a wonderful week. Patient has been having discharge.'

Mrs Cameron had had a total of 53 treatments by the time she testified at the Subcommittee hearing in Bracebridge in February 1939. A copy of her letter written to Dr Emma Carson, Los Angeles was submitted as an exhibit at the hearing.

To Dr E.M. Carson, M.D.
Hotel Hayward,
Los Angeles City, USA

18/8/37

Dear Dr Carson

I take pleasure in giving you briefly a statement of my condition before and since taking treatment (8 so far) from Rene M. Caisse of Bracebridge.

Intestinal trouble for years, the whole area from rectum to throat being affected. In September three years ago, I entered the Lockwood Clinic, Toronto. After X-ray and several consultations, they told me I had cancer of left kidney and, if not operated on, in six months it would be too late. My experience seemed to tell me that my chief trouble was at rectum and bowel. I sought further advice and was sent to the Western Hospital, Toronto. After many X-rays and consultations, time for my operation was set (they partially agreeing with diagnosis of the Lockwood Clinic), but I was then such a condition that my husband refused and took me home (I didn't care). I took the grape cure, other diets along with osteopathic treatments until June 1st of this year. I told the osteopath who was treating me that I was discouraged and that this sack of bowel was emptying about every three to four weeks – mucus, orange-coloured substance etc. He advised me to see Nurse Caisse of Bracebridge. After my first treatment this sack in bowel really did empty itself and had not refilled. I have also passed broken growth resembling pieces of sponge. Also just before my seventh treatment, I suffered great distress and soreness over the lower abdomen. I then passed a large, scab-like piece with much ropy colitis substance attached. There is a constant sloughing away of broken down tissue and ah, I am feeling so much better and have enjoyed this summer more than any in years. I am so happy to be feeling better and will certainly continue any treatments. I would do anything if other poor sufferers could have the help I believe Nurse Caisse could give them.

Yours very sincerely,
Isabel Cameron

BOWEL CANCER

Book One, Page 2, Case 2

Mr Archie Brooks, Age 52 years.

Physician: Dr K.H. Johnson and Dr R.H. Dillane, Powasssan, Ontario.
Diagnosis: malignancy of the bowel.
Patient had X-ray plates – malignancy of the bowel – North Bay General Hospital.

Copy of diagnosis:

TO WHOM IT MAY CONCERN:

This is to certify that we have examined Mr Archie Brooks of Loring and find that he has malignancy of the Bowel. This has been confirmed by X-ray examinations. This condition has emaciated this man so that he is unable to work in any way. Even if he were able, would not advise him to work on account of this condition.
Sincerely
Signed: K.H. Johnson M.D.
R.H. Dillane, Powassan

Remarks: first treatment by 'Essiac', 26 March 1937. Weight at that date, 148 1/2 lb. Patient at that time haemorrhaging freely, had distress in stomach, great pain in bowel, bloating from gas, soreness across bottom of stomach.
18 September 1937: patient feels well, still constipated, no bleeding for some time.
October 1938: patient very much improved, gain in weight, no obstruction in bowel, though not completely cured, is ready for an examination at any time. General condition very good, patient working every day.

Archie Brooks wrote to the Prime Minister of Ontario on Rene's behalf:

The Hon. Premier Hepburn   Loring, Ont.
House of Parliament
Toronto, Ont.

July 15th 1937

Dear Sir
    Having recently heard a rumour to the effect that there is a possibility of Miss Rene Caisse being prevented from using her remedy for cancer upon sufferers in Ontario, as one of those

sufferers, I desire to add my testimony to the evidence that Miss Caisse's cure is really a cure and to protest in the name of humanity against any movement on the part of the Medical Council or the Government that might interfere in any way with the good work she is doing.

The facts in my own case are as follows: It was February last that I was compelled to see the physician, Dr Dillane Jr of Powassan, for what I thought was some kind of stomach trouble. Dr Dillane sent me to St Joseph's Hospital in North Bay. I was X-rayed there and Dr Dillane advised me to get my X-ray plates from the hospital and go to Toronto for an operation. On questioning him, he told me the plates revealed Cancer of the Bowels. Dr Johnson, his assistant, agreed with the diagnosis and it seems to have been confirmed by the symptoms, obstruction and bleeding of the bowels.

On the way south, before calling in at the office of Dr Dillane in Powassan, I called upon a friend of mine, clergyman, who strongly advised me to see Miss Rene Caisse before having an operation. That was in April. I have been taking treatment from Miss Caisse ever since. My bowel trouble has almost cleared up and my bowels are almost normal, so far as the symptoms are concerned.

I am but one among many victims of cancer who could and, I hope, will testify to having been almost cured by Miss Caisse's remedy.

Surely before God, sir, you cannot allow this. I am not a physician, just a plain man who has suffered and is being healed, but the proof of the pudding is in the eating.

Sincerely yours
(Signed) Archie Brooks

LEG ULCERS

Book Three, Page 11, Case 9

Mrs George Keown, Age 66, Dwight, Ontario.

Physician: Dr McDonald, Huntsville, Ontario.
Diagnosis: ulcers of the leg of long standing.

Remarks: ulcers started 30 years ago. Patient had Dr McDonald of Huntsville operate on it. Twenty-five years ago Dr Hart operated on it, and again 16 years ago. Has been well until the summer of 1937 when patient came to Miss Caisse. Trouble in leg started as a milk leg. Patient has high blood pressure and nerves bad.

Patient started treatment by 'Essiac' 25 September 1937.
2 November 1937: patient feeling so much better, can walk better, eats and sleeps well and feels like living.
7 December 1937: patient says pain much less and leg healing fast. Says she used to spend sleepless nights with pain, now sleeps well. Had as many as 22 ulcers on her leg at one time, all healed now except one.

Mrs Keown wrote to Rene to verify her recovery:

February 16th 1938,
Dwight

Dear Miss Caisse

Got your card yesterday. Certainly use my name now and any other time you want to as regards your treatment.

Hoping you will forgive me for not writing to you before and letting you know about my leg. It is completely healed up for several weeks, no pain, no scab, only the scar remains. Have sent two or three letters to different papers letting the people know of the good results that I received from your treatment. Two weeks ago was rushed to the doctor's with a bad attack of appendix. Doctor wanted to operate the next day, however that spasm passed, am feeling very well again. While in the doctor's office, your name was mentioned. Dr White was quite interested and said he would like to see my leg if I didn't mind, and when he saw it, he said 'Miss Caisse has something I would like to get.' Also would I let Dr Evans see. I did want so bad for Dr Evans to see it. Dr White said he would ask him to come and have a look at it. When he came in, he never looked at it or never said a word, made no

comment whatever. However he didn't gain anything by it. So am going down sometime to see you. Will tell you the rest then.
Yours truly,
(Signed) Mrs G. Keown

GOITRE, STOMACH ULCERS, SORE ON LIP

Book Six, Page 6, Case 5

Mr J. Findlay, Age 36, Novar, Ontario.

Diagnosis: ulcers of the stomach, sore on lip, and goitre.
Remarks: patient had sore on lip seven months before coming for 'Essiac' treatment. Goitre was so large, patient could not button collar.

First treatment by 'Essiac' 6 July 1937.
3 September 1938: patient returned after lapse of no treatments for two months, with swelling in throat. Growth on lip and throat seemed affected. After seven treatments, swelling has decreased in size on side of neck and patient feels much better.
December 1938: patient has taken treatments at intervals since July 1937. Sore on lip has gone, patient has gained weight, can eat anything without distress and sleeps normally. Goitre has entirely disappeared.
Copy of letter written to Miss Caisse by Mr Findlay:

Novar, Dec. 6/38
To Miss Caisse Clinic,
Bracebridge

Madam – This is to say that I have had 22 treatments from June 16th 1937 to November 18th 1938 and my trouble improved in the meantime, and during the spell that the place was closed my lip was getting worse. I could not go during the winter for treatments, and in March the Clinic was closed till August 1938, when I again resumed treatments. The lip is improved and goitre had entirely disappeared. I am generally getting better all round, weight at beginning was 165 pounds and present weight 174 pounds. I feel confident that the treatments are helping my condition.

With best wishes to the Clinic, I remain,

Yours truly

(Signed) Jack Findlay

BREAST CANCER

Mrs Roy Coutts, Age 49.

August 1936: cancer of the right breast, hard nodular mass the size of a large apple, diagnosis confirmed by Dr Fraser Greig.

19 August 1936: first treatment at the Bracebridge Clinic, followed by five separate treatments. The growth had disappeared entirely after the sixth treatment.

21 November 1936: final treatment at Bracebridge Clinic.

Rene Caisse:

'I took this patient for Dr Greig, to give six treatments to localise the growth . . . Dr Greig intended to operate and {then} allow me to give six more treatments to prevent a recurrence.'

26 March 1937, Mrs C.:

'On August 19th 1936, I called at the clinic and . . . got my first treatment that day. In all I think it was 13 treatments {six by hypo and seven oral} when the growth was completely gone. So far there is no sign of it returning and I am enjoying perfect health at the age of fifty.'

WHEN PATIENTS DIED

Bereaved family members often wrote to thank Nurse Caisse for her help in caring for a loved one who died. One letter, signed by 20 relatives of a person who died of cancer, stated that the patient 'was a hopeless case, bleeding to death when you undertook to treat him. We consider that you prolonged his life, and for some time after he stopped taking treatments, he was without pain or bleeding. You benefited him greatly.'

The wife of a man with 'a huge carcinoma of the rectum with prostate involvement' who died after receiving a few

Essiac treatments (with radium treatments before Essiac) wrote: *'Many of the distressing features of that frightful disease were absent. One in particular was the unbearable odour present in advanced cases. In his case there was none.'*

An elderly female patient, hospitalised for the few remaining weeks of her life, developed a very severe, very painful shingles condition. It cleared up after being treated with Essiac. She no longer required any painkillers and died peacefully with a clear mind.

When the officials on the Cancer Commission Committee showed Rene a long list of patients believed to have died, she was able to prove that 75 per cent were still alive and well, while most of those who had died did not die as a direct result of their cancer.

Tea stories present

We are continually in receipt of letters and calls testifying to the efficacy of Essiac as the four-herb decoction in treating a variety of illnesses, including cancer. One lady reported: 'since I have been on Essiac, my rheumatoid arthritis has been very good. I can now get in and out of the bath without trouble. Also I could not open any bottles or cans but I do now.' Some people have reported having found great relief from irritable bowel syndrome after taking the tea, while one lady started taking Essiac for asthma and emphysema and wrote to us say she had had virtually no asthma attacks since then. She had changed her inhalers, but she was 'absolutely certain that Essiac is the prime reason for my improvement'. Another lady told us that she had suffered with eczema for 20 years. She had consulted skin specialists worldwide, costing a fortune in time and money. In less than a month of starting Essiac, her hands were clear, with just a few patches left on her legs, the condition continuing to improve as the summer months progressed, previously the most difficult time for her.

LIVER DISORDER

Mr L. Root sent us this report from the USA in January 2000:

'*Some years back, my wife and I were living in California and happened to hear a Mexican mom talking about her sick young daughter. Her little girl, about 12 years of age, had been taking antibiotics when something went wrong. Her liver was being damaged by whatever she was taking to the point that the doctors feared the liver would not survive. The total capacity of the liver function was below 30 per cent and failing. After putting the little girl on the liver donor list, the search for a new liver began.*

When we saw the girl, her face was bloated, discoloured and textured like a basketball. Her eyes had almost disappeared into her swollen head. She was in constant pain and could not go out in the daytime because the sun was a real bother to her. My wife thought perhaps the Essiac tea would ease some of the pain and the swelling, and the mother agreed to administer the tea to her daughter. We recommended one ounce, morning and night. After two weeks, the little girl looked a lot more normal and said she felt a lot better. Her Mom took her back to the doctor for a follow-up, and they were astounded to discover her liver function was improving rapidly! Last we heard, she was almost back to normal liver function, off the donor list and very happy to be back to living her life.

We have had friends who have had cancer and are now in complete remission, thanks to the tea. Also a friend whom we introduced to Essiac is no longer insulin dependent for diabetes. It's great stuff and so important to so many who had no hope'

HIV POSITIVE AND NON-HODGKINS LYMPHOMA

Miss R.B., UK, aged 29:

'*I was diagnosed HIV positive in January 1998 and diagnosed with Non-Hodgkins Lymphoma, centred in my pelvis and lumbar spine in the following May. Initially I resisted the antiviral medication for the HIV because I wasn't convinced by it. I have a nursing background and the "combination" therapy they were offering me was very new. No one knew enough about the long-term side effects.*

The treatment was all about timing. You have to take the doses regularly every 12 hours and the doctors said it could be disastrous if you missed one. I was absolutely terrified of the treatment and I felt too well to have it, except for some increasing pain in my lower back which had been diagnosed as sciatica. Eventually I had a scan which revealed a tumour in the spinal bone marrow. Biopsies confirmed the diagnosis – Non-Hodgkins Lymphoma.

The doctors wanted to put me straight on to chemotherapy and antiviral therapy simultaneously, in theory to cancel out the toxicity to my immune system during treatment. The problem is that 'well' HIV positive people on combination therapy can expect to be weak, vomiting, muscled-fatigued and very tired for six to eight weeks until their system gets used to the treatment.

I started on the treatment, having one drug administered by lumbar puncture and two or three more given intravenously. After the first session I vomited for two weeks. I had six sessions, once every three weeks over the next four months, and I vomited for two weeks out of every three. I would be just recovering when it was time to go back for the next session. The best of it was that the doctors told me that the cancer had probably gone after the first two doses but they were too scared not to give me the rest because no one had proved otherwise.

It was about this time I started taking Essiac combined with electro-crystal therapy and a complex supplement regime and, strangely enough, I did not lose any weight during the treatment period. I took multi antioxidants, multi-vitamins, essential fatty acids, blue–green algae, aloe vera, selenium, Siberian ginseng and cats claw, basically anything I thought would help.

The chemotherapy finished and I was still on the HIV antiviral treatment. I felt very weak but just starting to build myself up again when I went down with shingles–herpes zoster around my stomach. Fortunately I was only ill for about 10 days so I was lucky.

My cancer check-up was due at the end of the year in December. The results were not good. The cancer had recurred and it was worse. I was referred to a consultant haemotologist for advice about more chemotherapy but there was some doubt as to whether my immune system could take any more toxic treatment. I got the feeling that the doctors thought I was finished and they were backing off. I didn't agree and made an appointment with my electro-crystal therapist for another scan. He didn't agree with the doctors either.

My sister came with me to see the haemotologist and, while we were sitting in the consulting room, the oncologist came in to tell us that the radiologist had taken another look at the scans and decided that what they had seen was not a recurrence of the cancer but probably scar tissue as a result of the healing process. It was such a relief.

I continued with the combination, antiviral therapy and the various supplements, making a few changes such as taking out the ginseng and the cats claw. But I kept up with the Essiac for the HIV and as a preventative to stop the lymphoma returning. My T cell count was steadily climbing, the viral load was undetectable and I was making good progress. I had been smoking cannabis for years and by April 1999 I felt healthy enough to give it up. I had used it a lot while I was on chemotherapy to help with the nausea and the stress but I was afraid of becoming addicted.

I started two courses in complementary health in September 1999 and as a result of what I was beginning to learn, I made a conscious decision to stop having the combination therapy. Everyone thought I was mad, except my partner (who is HIV negative) and my homeopath. Friends and family generally said nothing but had their reservations. The doctors openly tried to dissuade me but I was determined. I knew that if I didn't try it, I would always regret it.

As it was, I felt so much better in myself once I was off the treatment. My confidence came back and I got a great sense of freedom and empowerment. I was clearer, less "foggy" and no longer nauseous. The pains in my feet and the numbness in my arms went away and the lypodystrophy condition was no longer progressive, beginning very slowly to reverse over the next few months. Lypodystrophy is a fairly common side effect of the antiviral treatment, affecting more women than men, and clinics have been set up specifically to deal with this problem. It involves fat redistribution in the body, in this case concentrating all the fat on the torso at the expense of the rest of the body. Over a year after stopping the treatment, I am still round in the middle but my arms and legs have filled out a little and I look more in proportion again.

Since then there has been steady progress. My viral load has fluctuated, which is only to be expected, usually triggered by stress. When my sister had an accident and broke her back, the viral load went off the scale at over 1,000,000 copies/mL, falling to 128,000 copies/mL as she got better, not undetectable but much improved. My T cell count had been fairly constant at 100 and fell to 70 before stabilising.

I religiously keep up with all my supplements and my Essiac as a means of keeping well and I keep myself fit by doing yoga and Tai chi. I drink three litres of mineral water every day with the occasional glass of red wine. I only had one very mild cold during last winter's flu epidemic, my studies are going very well and my partner has been an absolute star, supporting me and helping me all the way through.

I would recommend anyone who is HIV positive to take Essiac because you need every available force to boost the immune system. HIV-related cancers are increasing and I believe Essiac is a useful, two-in-one ally, something positive that's fighting on your side of the fence.'

PROSTATE CANCER
Mr C.F., UK, aged 59:

'I was diagnosed with prostate cancer on November 26th 1999 after I started having problems passing water, sometimes getting up two or three times every night. I was beginning to get a lot of pain as well on days after I came back from working on my fishing boat and lifting the nets and the weights. I went to my local doctor and he gave me a blood test. He said, "if you don't hear anything in the next few days, you're all right." When the results of the test came back, my

PSA count was 65.8. This time the doctor said, 'You've got the Big C. You'd better go and see a specialist.'

I was down at the hospital a week or so later for another blood test, biopsies and a bone scan. By then the PSA count was 68.5 and rising. The bone scan came back clear but they said I had a large, metastatic tumour. They didn't recommend surgery because they said I might only have a 6 per cent chance of recovery. They put me on a hormone suppressant and gave me an appointment date for two months later.

By this time I was in a lot of pain. I couldn't sit down. I had to lie down all the time just to try and be comfortable. The worst thing was that I didn't feel supported. There was no advice about diet or anything like that. I was just left to fend for myself. I went out for a drive, feeling terrible. As I was driving down the road, I noticed the door open in one of our local health shops. I parked the car and went in. A man asked me if I wanted any help, and I told him I had just been diagnosed with inoperable cancer. He recommended I try Essiac, along-side the hormone treatment. Ten days later I was able to sit down again without any pain, and people didn't even think I had cancer. I passed a much darker-coloured urine for five to six weeks: I was passing pieces of creamy-greenish coloured growth from my back passage and an unusual sticky substance started coming down my nose.

Six weeks later my PSA count was down to 7.9, and that's when all the trouble started because the doctors wanted me to have radiotherapy. I was supposed to have 20 treatments of between 10 and 15 minutes a time. Now I was worried about this because I had heard of other people having a really bad time after they had radiotherapy. It might have helped the cancer but it messed up everything else. I didn't want that. When I refused to have it the radiotherapy consultant told me I wouldn't be offered the treatment again. My local doctor talked him into putting me back on the list but it didn't make any difference. I was not going to have radiotherapy, not unless my PSA count started going up again and there was nothing else.

I decided I would have to look after myself. I changed my diet, giving up milk and red meat. I started buying all organic food, I don't smoke or drink and I gave up using the microwave. I stopped buying the Essiac product from the health shop because it was too expensive and I started making up my own. The quality was consistently better and it cost a fraction of the price.

I have been taking Essiac continually since the diagnosis and I started using the diluted Sheep sorrel solution as an enema twice a week from April 2000. At first the enemas made my back passage feel sore, so I stopped using them for a couple of weeks and then started again. This time I found I was getting a lot of heat right up my back to my neck after using the enema. I had always had a lot of pain in my back and in my neck, but that's gone now. I used to get blinding headaches, but not any more. I had suffered with haemorrhoids since I was a teenager, and now they've gone as well. I used to have a very sensitive stomach, I couldn't eat very spicy food and not a lot of vegetables. Now I can eat just about anything. And when I wore the skin off my knee under my oilskins out at sea, I soaked a piece of Kleenex in the Sheep sorrel solution and held it against the wound twice a day for only two days and it healed completely.

When I saw the consultant again four months later in June, he told me the prostate was back to normal and they couldn't see any sign of the tumour on the scans. The PSA count was 2.8. He told me to carry on with the hormone treatment and to see him again in six months' time.

I've been varying the Essiac treatment. I've been taking the medicine all the time, taking the 30 ml dose once daily at night for three weeks of every month and taking the same dose morning and night for one week in every month. I used the enema once every third day at night for a month. Then I gave it a break and started again, using it once a week. I vary the enema treatment depending on how I feel. If I don't feel so good, I do it twice a week instead of just once. And I take breaks from using it, just relying on the oral Essiac to do the job. *My energy levels are good, my appetite's good and everything's back to normal. I regularly go through the night without getting up.*

I wish I wasn't taking the hormone treatment because I'm not sure about the side effects, and I'm not sure the doctors know either. One doctor told me that it might only work for 18 months at the most. I'm not even sure that I need it now because I'm doing far better than they said I would. I'm going to be taking the Essiac until I drop. I'm helping all sorts of people now. I've seen them sent home to die, go on to the Essiac and then they're dancing. They're responding within eight to 10 days and they're doing well. One lady has a huge cancer entwined around her sciatic nerve. When I first met her, she could hardly walk and she was in a lot of pain. Now she's walking over to my house and going to the local cancer support group. Another lady with leukaemia went from 50 per cent cancer cells in her blood down to 2 per cent to totally clear. Results like that make it all worth while.'

OVARIAN CANCER
Gianine O'Shea, UK:

'I'm still here and still fighting ovarian cancer. I have had to deal with pain since I wrote my last report for Essiac Essentials, *but not because of the cancer. I have kept the cancer mostly under control with a careful balance of diet, Essiac and for a while with Hydrazine sulphate. My problems have occurred as a result of past chemotherapy and damaging surgical treatment.*

If I could go back to the first days of my diagnosis with the knowledge I have now, I would do it so differently. I would never have allowed myself to be persuaded to start on chemotherapy and I would have asked so many more questions before I had surgery. It seems that when you start on the chemicals, you're stuck with them, like I am. The brave ones who say 'no' right from the start are the ones who are surviving. I know one woman with breast cancer who refused all conventional treatment seven years ago. She went straight on to a herbal mixture which she thinks was based on Essiac. Her herbalist was charging her a lot of money for the treatment and refused to tell her exactly what was in the mixture. Whatever it was, it worked and the tumour gradually shrank away.

Patients like her must be studied. No one studies the survivors, the ones who do it with diet and alternative therapies. They should be properly monitored and given access to regular blood testing or scanning, whatever they decide they need. The trouble is that there are no guidelines for people who want to manage their cancer themselves. There are plenty of books about alternative treatments and plenty of people wanting to take your money, but there is no time to try all the different therapies and find out which one is the best. I have dabbled in all sorts of things over the last four years, but I would have preferred to have kept to one or two things right from the beginning. I know that Essiac helps me and I know that a combination of Essiac and hydrazine sulphate has helped me. The trouble is that the doctors fill us up with all the bad stuff first, leaving no room for the good stuff. They filled me up with something alien, and I don't know enough about my body to be able to judge exactly what is happening.

Since I have survived well past my "sell-by" date, I have become a veteran, I'm not classifiable and everything's done on "compassionate grounds". If I have a pain, it's always "expected". There's no encouragement. No aches and pains in my body are allowed to be anything but a direct result of the cancer. It took months to persuade the doctors that I needed a course of anti-inflammatory drugs rather than morphine for the pain resulting from surgery I had almost a year ago. But being a veteran does have some advantages. I can try any treatment I want to. No one bothers to tell me I mustn't do something because it might be detrimental to my health. In their opinion, "health" is something I don't have any more.

During April 2000, I was in a pretty bad way. I had been losing blood and mucus from my back passage from secondary tumours in the bowel and in a continual state of partial blockage, with all the related discomfort and pain. It was getting almost impossible to eat without nausea and pain, and I was losing a lot of weight. Like most cancer patients, I will try anything someone else has proved to work. There's a lot written about various treatments but not a lot of actual proof. And I need proof. I decided to stop taking the hydrazine sulphate and I tracked down another survivor to see what she had been doing. The Sheep sorrel enema was an option I decided to try. As far as I was concerned I had nothing to lose.

I used the enema once every three days for two weeks. I had to hang myself upside down for 20 minutes every time to make sure that all the herb solution managed to trickle down to where it was most needed. After the first week, I noticed a change. There was still a lot of pain but something had changed. I had my first dose of Taxol at the end of the second week. The next day, the tumour burst and I passed a lot of dark, smelly stuff that definitely was not faeces.

Within a few days, I stopped passing blood and mucus, the pain went away and I was able to eat normally again. I had another dose of Taxol, more to keep the doctors happy than anything else, and I had virtually no side effects from the chemotherapy, just losing most of my hair, as I expected, but otherwise feeling fine. My CA125 count was back down to 10.

My job is to get this disease sorted out. I recognise wisdom in myself now, and I have touched a happiness I didn't know before. I have so much support from my family and friends, people don't shy away because I happen to have cancer. I know it was all meant to be, and every experience I go through helps me to help someone else maybe to do it better and get it right. Because everyone believes they can win the lottery, but no one stops to think they have a much greater chance of getting cancer the way life is now.

If you don't have cancer, take intelligent precautions. You clean your teeth to stop cavities but you never think about cancer prevention until you've got it. And if you do get it, start with the good stuff. Sort out your diet, take your Essiac and start asking a lot of questions. Look at the alternative therapies available and find out which ones might be best for you. Don't be afraid to take charge of your own life with your cancer.

Don't be afraid to do it how you want to do it. There are plenty of other people out there feeling just like you do. You might not know any of them, but they're there and determined to sort themselves out and get it right. Always remember, you are not alone.'

Notes on the 1939 Cancer Commission Hearings

*T*he patients' statements compiled at the Subcommittee hearing in Bracebridge in February 1939 and at the 4 July hearing in Toronto, including statements made under oath by the nurse herself, represent the most accurate, official record of Rene Caisse's work at the Bracebridge Clinic. Of the 66 statements taken, 34 were almost duplicated as 17 patients volunteered to testify at both hearings. The testimonies from the February hearing are largely more detailed because the commissioners had allocated more time to be made available for hearing the witnesses.

When estimating a patient's recovery time scales, allowance must be made for the nine periods between 1937 and 1941 when the clinic was closed, listed as follows:

1   8 February 1937–5 April 1937 after Rene collapsed from exhaustion and went to Michigan to stay with her sister until she was well enough to open the clinic again.
2   April 1937, third week, closed briefly when Rene experienced some minor heart problems. She went to Toronto to stay with another of her sisters.
3   29 July–7 August 1937, closed.
4   October 1937, closed for two weeks after Dr Emma Carson's extended visit during August and September of that year.
5   22 December 1937, closed for three weeks for Christmas.

6   Early 1938, the clinic was closed for several weeks, and due to be reopened on 25 March, but it remained closed while Rene rested in Florida during April 1938 after her Bill was rejected by the Ontario Parliament.

7   23 May 1938–5 August 1938, closed for 10 weeks.

8   22 December 1938–3 February 1939, closed for six weeks, reopening in time for the Subcommittee hearing.

9   End of January 1940, closed for some weeks. The clinic finally closed in January 1941.

Of the patients:

Mrs Annie Rudd was a professional nurse.

Mrs Elsie Graham testified as having been treated with douches as well as the oral and injectable therapies.

Mr Sam Holingshead was treated once a month over a period of 21 months for stomach cancer.

Mr John McNee was treated with the oral medicine and with the Sheep sorrel solution topically over a six-month period for his cancer of the lip. He received no injections during that time.

Mr Robert Caldwell was treated daily by injections administered by his wife for cancer of the lower rectum, reducing to twice weekly as his condition improved.

Mr Lorne Fraser was treated regularly over two years for his cancer of the mouth, but his condition reverted during clinic closure times.

Mrs Edith Guppy was treated 25 times over a period of 15 months for her skin cancer, by injection in either arm, orally and the Sheep sorrel solution applied topically.

Mrs Gertrude Scott received 40 treatments over 11 months for stomach ulcers, probably brought on by her extremely stressed condition after a sexually abusive experience in childhood.

Mrs A.G. Cameron was treated 60 times over an 18-month period by injection and with the oral medicine for kidney cancer. She reported the 'chills and fever' sensation lasting as long as 24 hours after treatment.

Mr William O'Brien's testimony was dismissed because he had been diagnosed as having 'benign atrophy of the prostate'.

Commissioner Wallace told him: 'we are only dealing with cancer cases'.

Mr John Tynan was treated by injection 27 times over 10 months, and said that he had begun to feel better after the first four days.

Mrs Clara Thornbury had been carried into the clinic for her first treatments and saw a great improvement in her cancer of the stomach condition after three treatments.

Mr Brodie, officiating at the February hearing, refused to believe William Giles had face cancer if he chewed tobacco.

Mr J.W. Vanclieff was treated by injection in the leg once a month for cancer of the rectum.

Mrs May Henderson passed pieces of tumour with each monthly menstrual period for more than two and a half years.

Mrs Eliza Veitch was treated only with the oral remedy for 13 months for cancer of the womb. She remarked that she thought the oral treatment was slower than the injectable therapy. She showed no reaction until after the eighth treatment, which she described as a 'bad' reaction, and then she began to improve.

Mrs Elsie Graham's diagnosis of cancer of the uterus was disputed at the February hearing.

Rachel Whitmore received 50 treatments by injection over 18 months for her cancer of the uterus and breast, a total of 24 in one arm, 25 in the other arm and one in the leg.

Mr Stanley Thurston's cancer of the rectum broke up and came away in pieces after 12 months of treatment.

Mrs Sarah Tibbel's cancer had metastasised with a growth on her forehead. She began treatment on 5 August 1938, injections + oral + the Sheep sorrel solution applied topically. The growth came off in her hand after 10 treatments.

It is unclear whether Mrs Nellie McVittie actually had cancer of the womb. Whatever her condition, a Mrs Gladys Partlett recalled Nellie being carried into the clinic, haemorrhaging badly, in 1936. Dr Dale (from Sudbury) believed Nellie had cancer of the uterus and the neck of the womb. Prior to Essiac treatments, the neck of the womb had been cauterised, causing heavy and prolonged bleeding for six weeks after treatment. Nellie's condition had been becoming steadily more serious over the previous winter. After the Essiac treatments began in May 1936, the bleeding stopped within 24 hours and her monthly periods normalised after two months. Nellie died in 1992, aged 98.

When Rene was working at the Brusch Medical Center in 1959, Dr McClure asked her to write to 26 of her former patients to find out how many were still alive at that time. Twenty-two patients signed and returned the 'To Whom This May Concern' letter, assuring the nurse that they were well and free from cancer.

In 1976, 13 former patients replied to a similar letter. Of these, Mrs Guppy was now 61, nine others were in their seventies, two were in their eighties and Clara Thornbury was in her 91st year. Fred Walker, who used to bring Rene beautiful black cherries from the Niagara fruit belt (he lived in Beamsville), was 87 when he died in 1991.

Subcommittee Hearing, Bracebridge, Ontario, 3/4 February 1939

No.	Name	Cancer	No.Treatments	Treatment Time	Age/1939	Age/1959	Age/1977	Book No.	Case No.
1	George Bruce*	Lip/Cheek	no record	8 mths	61 years			4	4
2	Mrs E. Forsythe	Uterus	no record	12 mths	55 years	78 years		5	4
3	S.J. Reynolds	Mouth	no record	24 mths	no record			no record	no record
4	W.J. O'Brien	None – case dismissed			61 years			4	12
5	J.W. Vanclieff*	Rectum	no record	12 mths	no record			3	17
6	Mrs E. Stewart	Uterus	52	24 mths	53 years	76 years		5	17
7	R.J. Wolfenden*	Rectum	57	10 mths		no record		3	19
8	R.G. Long*	Rectum/Prostate	54	22 mths		60 years		5	8
9	Mrs Annie Rudd	Rectum/Cervix	23	7 mths	43 years			no record	no record
10	Alex McDougall*	Stomach	42	14 mths	76 years			3	11
11	Walter Lawson	Back of Ear	30	no record	74 years			2	20
12	Mrs C. Thornbury*	Stomach	55	18 mths	52 years	75 years	91 years	1	14
13	W.J. Durnford	Rectum	7	2 mths	no record			no record	no record
14	Thomas Windette	Lower Lip	no record	6 mths	69 years			4	19
15	Elsie Graham*	Uterus	no record	21mths	47 years			1	4
16	Sam Holingshead	Stomach	21	21mths	65 years			4	9
17	John McNee*	Lip	no record	6 mths	67 years	91 years		2	2
18	Herbert Rawson	Rectum	no record	11mths	48 years	63 years		3	15
19	Robert Caldwell	Lower Rectum	multiple	15 mths	62 years			4	5
20	Mrs D. Heinbecker	Uterus	approx. 40	5 Mths & 3 mths	56 years			3	8
21	Lorne Fraser*	Mouth	approx. 70	24mths	57 years			no record	no record
22	William R. Giles*	Face	20	14mths	no record			no record	no record
23	Miss A. Rumball*	Breast	40–50	18mths	35 years	57 years	75 years	2	27
24	Mrs Edith Guppy*	Skin (Hand)	25	15 mths	21 years	43 years	61 years	1	6
25	Gertrude Scott	Stomach Ulcers	40	11 mths	no record			no record	no record
26	William Peacock	Lip	59	22 mths	43 years			no record	no record
27	Hattie Wurts*	Cervix	no record	9 mths	no record			3	20
28	Mrs A.G. Cameron	Kidney	60	18 mths	56 years			3	5
29	Mrs R. Allman	Stomach	30	6 mths	65 years			4	1
30	Mrs Minnie Norris	Bowel+Diabetes	23	9 mths	64 years			1	11

* indicates patients who testified at both February and July hearings.

Cancer Commision Hearing, Toronto, 4 July 1939

No.	Name	Cancer	No. Treatments	Treatment Time	Age/1939	Age/1959	Age/1977	Book No.	Case No.
1	E.R. Rose	Nose	no record	6 mths	no record			no record	no record
2	Newman R. Craig	Prostrate	6	no record	no record			no record	no record
3	Edith Guppy	Skin(Hand)	25	15 mths	21 years	43 years	61 years	1	6
4	John Tynan	Rectum	27	10 mths	69 years			3	16
5	W. Hampson	Lip	8 or 9	no record	34 years			1	8
6	Annie Bonar	Arm/Uterus	weekly	20 mths	53 years			3	4
7	Emma Forsythe	Uterus	no record	12 mths	55 years	78 years		5	4
8	Mrs. C. Thornbury	Stomach	55	18 mths	52 years	75 years	91 years	1	14
9	Peter Hanon	Bowel	no record	14 mths	no record			no record	no record
10	William Giles	Face	20	4 mths	no record			no record	no record
11	John H. Loughlin	Oesophagus	no record	17 mths	no record			no record	no record
12	Nellie McVittie	Uterus	no record	12 mths	42 years	65 years	82 years	5	12
13	J.W. Vanclieff	Rectum		28 mths	no record			3	17
14	May Henderson	Breast/Uterus	65	22 mths	41 years	63 years	81 years	1	9
15	R.G. Long	Rectum/Prostate	54	7 mths	60 years			5	8
16	Annie Rudd	Rectum/Cervix	23	18 mths	43 years			no record	no record
17	George Mahon	Bowel	irregular	14 mths	62 years			5	10
18	Alex McDougall	Stomach	42	11 mths	76 years			3	11
19	Rebecca Miller	Bowel	no record	8 mths	71 years			no record	no record
20	George Bruce	Lip/Cheek	no record	24mths	61 years			4	4
21	Lorne Fraser	Mouth	approx.70	no record	57 years			no record	no record
22	Herbert Rawson	Rectum	no record		48 years	63 years		3	15
23	Hattie Wurts	Cervix	no record	9 mths	no record			3	20
24	Tony Baziuk	Lip	5	6 weeks	38 years	61 years	79 years	1	1
25	Augusta Douglas	Cervix	no record	11 mths	no record			6	4
26	Eliza Veitch	Uterus	no record	13 mths	55 years	77 years		5	19
27	Elsie Graham	Uterus		21 mths	47 years			1	4
28	Elizabeth Stewart	Uterus	52	15 mths	53 years	76 years		5	17
29	Laura Swayze	Breast	no record		no record	lived another 25 years			
30	Wilson Hammel	Rectum	50–70	30 mths	50 years	74 years		1	5
31	John McNee	Lip	no record	7 mths	67 years	91 years		2	2

Cancer Commission Hearing, Toronto 4 July 1939

No.	Name	Cancer	No. Treatments	Treatment Time	Age/1939	Age/1959	Age/1977	Book No.	Case No.
32	Rachel Whitmore	Breast/Uterus	50 (hypo)	18 mths	no record			no record	no record
33	Stanley Thurston	Rectum	no record	12 mths	no record			no record	no record
34	Sarah Tibble	Uterus/Vagina	10	12 mths	55 years	79 years		no record	no record
35	Alma Rumball	Breast	40–50	18 mths	35 years	57 years	75 years	2	27
36	Richard Wolfenden	Rectum	57	10 mths	no record			3	19
37	Dr. Benjamin Leslie Guyatt's Testimony on Behalf of Miss Rene Caisse								

Appendix II

Herb Analysis

This appendix gives technical details of 15 herbs featured in this book, beginning with the basic four-herb ingredients for Essiac – Sheep sorrel, Burdock, Slippery elm and Turkey rhubarb – and then listing others, both herbs that were included in or have been suspected of being a part of Rene Caisse's secret eight-herb formula and others. For each herb the table shows active ingredients, antioxidant properties and other vitamins, anti-free radical and other minerals, anti-cancer activity and energy type plus pH values.

Herb	Active ingredients	Antioxidant properties	Other vitamins	Anti-free radical minerals	Other minerals	Anti-cancer activity	Energy + pH value (decoction)
SHEEP SORREL whole herb (*Rumex acetosella*)	Aloe emodin; organic acids: citric, malic, oxalic tannic, tartaric	Vit. A, C+P, E carotenoids + para-aminobenzoic acid; chlorophyls	Vit B complex D, K, U	Copper, manganese, zinc	Calcium, chlorine iron, magnesium, silicon, sulphur, trace iodine	High as whole herb	Bitter, cool pH 4.5
Sheep sorrel seeds	As whole herb +	Vit. E	Vit. B complex pangamic acid, amygdalin	Manganese			
Sheep sorrel roots	As whole herb + anthracenocides; anthraquinones: chrysophanol, emodin, physcion, quercitin						
BURDOCK root (*Arctium lappa*)	Inulin – to 45% (1st yr) mucilage – to 12%; sugars, benzaldehyde, bitter glycosides: arctiopicrin, lappin; flavanoids inc. arctiin; some phyto-oestrogen activity	Vit. A, C+P, E; tannins	Vit. B complex	Zinc, manganese, selenium, trace copper	High-chromium, iron, magnesium, silicon, tin; aluminium, niacin, cobalt, phosphorus, potassium, silicon, sodium, trace calcium, sulphur	Noted	Bitter, cool, slightly sweet pH 6
Burdock seeds	Flavanoids inc. arctiin, arctigenin; gobosterin; essential oil; fatty oil						Less bitter

Herb	Active ingredients	Antioxidant properties	Other vitamins	Anti-free radical minerals	Other minerals	Anti-cancer activity	Energy + pH value (decoction)
SLIPPERY ELM inner bark (*Ulmus rubra*)	Mucilage – 20–30% organic acid – gallic phenols; sugars; starch 8–21%; beta-sitosterol; polysaccharides; carbohydrates; high in dietary fibre	Vit. A, C+P, tannins	Vit. B complex (high), K	Manganese, selenium, trace zinc	Calcium, niacin (high), chromium, tin, cobalt, magnesium, potassium, sodium; trace aluminium, iron, phosphorus, silicon	Some	Sweet, neutral pH 7
TURKEY RHUBARB root (*Rheum palmatum*)	Anthraquinone glycosides as: rhein, chrysphanic acid, rheochrysidin; aloe-emodin; catechins; organic acids: gallic, oxalic, malic, tannic	Vit. A, C+P	Vit. B complex (partial)	Copper, manganese, zinc	Calcium, chlorine, iodine, iron, silicon, magnesium, sodium, phosphorus, sulphur, potassium	Noted	Bitter, cool pH 5
JUNIPER berries (*Juniperus communis*)	Volatile oils – pinene, myrcene, sabinene, terpinene, camphene, thujone; sugars; flavanoids; resin; gallotannins	Vit. A, trace C+P tannins	Not noted	Selenium (high), manganese, trace zinc	Chromium, cobalt, tin, calcium, iron, silicon, aluminium magnesium, niacin, potassium, thiamine, trace phosphorus, sodium, riboflavin	Noted	Bitter, hot pH 7

Herb	Active ingredients	Antioxidant properties	Other vitamins	Anti-free radical minerals	Other minerals	Anti-cancer activity	Energy + pH value (decoction)
PRICKLY ASH bark (*Zanthoxylum americanum/Z. clavaherculis*)	Volatile oil; gum; acrid resin; alkaloids: berberine, chelerythrine, lauroflorine, nitidine, magnoflorine	Not noted	Not noted	Not noted	Not noted	Noted	Spicy, warm pH 6.5
berries	Greater stimulant properties than bark						
URVA URSI leaves (*Arctostaphylos uva-ursi*)	Phenolic glycosides phenols; hydroquinone, glycosides (5–18%): methyl-arbutin, arbutin, ericolin; allantoin; flavanoids (quercetin); organic acids: egallic, gallic, quinic; ursone	Vit A (high) C+P; tannins (6–7%)	Not noted	Manganese, selenium, trace zinc	Aluminium, iron, calcium, chromium, cobalt, magnesium, niacin, potassium, sodium, thiamine; trace phosphorus, tin, riboflavin	Enhances cytotoxic activity	Bitter, cold, astringent pH 8
BLOODROOT root (*Sanguinaria candensis*)	Alkaloids: sanguinarine, sanguidimerine, chlolerythrine, protopine, copticine, berberine; red resin; tannic acid as in Tormentil	Not noted	Not noted	Not noted	Not noted	Possible	Bitter, hot **classified unsafe/ toxic** pH 5.5

Herb	Active ingredients	Antioxidant properties	Other vitamins	Anti-free radical minerals	Other minerals	Anti-cancer activity	Energy + pH value (decoction)
BALSAM OF PERU (*Myroxylon pereirae*)	Cinnamein; gum benzoin; peruviol; vanillin; cinnamic acid; coumarin (fruits)	Not noted	Not noted	Not noted	Not noted	Not noted	Warm, aromatic pH value not noted
CLEAVERS (*Galium aparine*)	Coumarin glycosides, inc. asperuloside; anthraquinone galiosin; organic acids inc. citric	Tannins	Not noted	Not noted	Not noted	Not noted	Bitter, cool pH 7
GOLD THREAD (*Coptis trifolia, var. groenlandica*)	Alkaloids: berberine (highest percentage in any known plant); coptine; albumen	Not noted	Not noted	Not noted	Not noted	Not noted	Bitter, cold pH value not noted
PERIWINKLE (*Vinca major, Vinca minor*)	Alkaloids: vincamine, reserpine	Tannins	Not noted	Not noted	Not noted	Possible (noted in Madagascan periwinkle, *Catharanthus roseus*)	Bitter, cool pH 7.5

Herb	Active ingredients	Antioxidant properties	Other vitamins	Anti-free radical minerals	Other minerals	Anti-cancer activity	Energy + pH value (decoction)
RED CLOVER (*Trifolium pratense*)	Glycosides: phenolic (inc. trifolin) & cyanogenic; salycylic acid; coumarins, inositol, daldzein, genistein; isoflavone biochanin A; uzarin; phyto-oestrogen: coumerol	Vit. A, C+P flavonoids	Vit. B complex	Copper, manganese, selenium, zinc	Biotin, chlorine, chromium, magnesium	Noted	Sweet, salty, cooling, oestrogenic pH 6
WATERCRESS (*Rorippa nasturtium-aquaticum*)	Mustard oil glycosides	Vit. C+P (high) A, E	Vit. B2	Copper, manganese, zinc	Calcium, iodine, iron phosphorus, sulphur	Not noted	Spicy, bitter, warm pH 7
YELLOW DOCK (*Rumex crispus*)	Anthraquinones; anthraquinone glycosides based on emodin and chrysophenic acid; phenols and phenolic glycosides; rumicin; chrysarobin; oxalic acid bio-available source of iron	Vit. A, C+P (high) tannins	Not noted	Selenium, magnesium, trace zinc	High: thiamine, iron, magnesium, phosphorus, aluminium, calcium, riboflavin, tin; niacin, potassium, cobalt, silicon, sodium, trace chromium	Not noted	Bitter, cool pH 6.5

Glossary of Terms

adenocarcinoma A malignant tumour originating in glandular tissue.

AIDS Acquired immune deficiency syndrome: a disorder that can suddenly alter the body's ability to defend itself as the AIDS virus invades the T cells and multiplies. The immune system breaks down, leading to overwhelming infection and/or cancer and possibly death.

alcohols A large group of compounds often found in volatile oils.

alkaloids Compounds containing a nitrogen atom. Alkaloids are usually present in plants as groups of chemicals. Their physical effects include killing pain, poisoning and causing hallucinations.

alteratives Treat toxicity of the blood, infections, arthritis, cancer and skin eruptions. They help the body to assimilate nutrients and eliminate metabolic waste products. The accompanying properties of an alterative herb are matched with the specific nature of the condition being treated.

anthraquinones Glycoside compounds that produce dyes and purgatives.

antibody Any of various proteins generated in the blood to neutralise foreign substances and so provide immunity against further infections.

antigen Any substance that stimulates the production of an antibody when introduced into the body.

antioxidants May alter the rate of occurrence of cancer and its subsequent growth through their action as anti-carcinogens,

161

alleviating and protecting against damaging free radicals or reacting with their by-products.

antispasmodic Compound or substance that eases or prevents spasms.

astringent Describes the binding action of many herbal remedies on mucous membranes and exposed tissues, providing an impenetrable barrier to most infective organisms and many toxins.

B cell As a B lymphocyte, an immune system cell that circulates in the blood stream. Once activated, B cells divide and differentiate into plasma cells, secreting large amounts of antibody to the antigen that stimulated the immune response.

bitters Herbs containing a range of chemicals that have a bitter taste. Some are useful as appetite stimulants, some as anti-inflammatories, others as relaxants.

blood count The number of red and white blood cells and platelets in a sample of blood.

CA125 Tumour marker blood test specific to ovarian cancer; elevation initially indicates immune response.

carbohydrates The most common plant carbohydrates are the nutritionally important sugars, starches and cellulose.

carcinogen Any agent that causes cancer.

carcinoma Any of a large variety of malignant tumours derived from epithelial cells covering the surface of a tissue.

cardio-active glycosides Substances having a strong effect on the heart (*digitalis*).

carotene Is converted into vitamin A in the body from the yellow pigment in the form of alpha-, beta- and gamma carotene.

CAT scan Computerised axial tomography scan using X-rays and a computer to detect abnormalities in the organs of the body; the results are limited in comparison with an MRI scan.

cell proliferant A substance that acts to reproduce or produce new cells rapidly and repeatedly.

coumarins Glycoside compounds responsible for the 'new-mown hay' smell of many grasses.

decoction A preparation made by boiling remedies in water.

demulcents Remedies that are primarily soothing in effect, characteristically serving to enhance associated healing or astringent properties.

diaphoretic Inducing perspiration.

diuretic A substance that causes an increased output of urine.

DNA Deoxyribonucleic acid, the substance found in the nucleus of all cells and genetically codes the amino acids and their peptide chain, determining the type of life form into which the cell will develop.

douche Washing out a body cavity or an opening by a stream of water or other fluid, often used to describe a vaginal wash-out for women.

dysphagia Difficulty in swallowing.

enema The introduction of fluid into the rectum for therapeutic purposes.

enzymes Specific protein catalysts that increase the chemical reaction time in the body without being consumed.

essential fatty acids As in linoleic acid, linolenic acid and arachidonic acid – deficiency shows as scaly dermatitis.

expectorant A substance that assists in the removal of sticky, mucoid sputum from the bronchial tubes.

flavonoid glycosides Common group of plant chemicals named for their yellow colour. Name derived from the Latin *flavus*, meaning yellow. Actions include diuretics, circulatory stimulants and anti-spasmodics.

free radicals Activated and hugely destructive molecules routinely produced in small amounts during the normal cell cycle and generated in excessive amounts by chemotherapy and radiotherapy. Free radicals are associated with many damaging conditions, including cancer, radiation sickness and rheumatoid arthritis.

giardia A parasitic protozoan (*Giardia lamblia*) causing infestation of the small intestine with characteristic bloating feelings, diarrhoea and nausea.

glioblastoma multiforme Astrocytoma grade IV. Diffusely invasive of normal brain cells, so tumour cells are usually left behind during surgery.

glucoside A specific sugar related to a product of glucose.

glycosides Common plant chemicals consisting of molecules made up of two sections, one being a sugar.

gulag A forced labour camp or prison in Russia, particularly for political prisoners.

HIV Human immunodeficiency virus, causing AIDS.

hyper- As in high capacity.

hypo- As in low capacity.

hypoxia Deficiency of oxygen in the tissues.

immune system A combination of cells and proteins working together to fight harmful bacteria and viruses. The well-being of the liver, spleen, thymus, bone marrow and lymphatic system are all vitally important to the immune system's normal function.

immunosuppression As in an immunosuppressive drug: to suppress the natural immune response of an organism to an antigen.

infusion A preparation made by steeping remedies in hot water.

laparotomy Surgical incision into the abdominal wall, either to determine diagnosis or as a prelude to further surgery.

leucocyte Any of the white or colourless nucleated cells occurring in the blood, also called a 'white blood cell'.

leukaemia Cancer of the lymph glands and bone marrow resulting in the overproduction of white blood cells (related to Hodgkins disease).

lymph A clear fluid flowing through the lymph vessels, which is collected from the tissues throughout the body in order to nourish tissue cells and return waste matter to the blood stream via the veins.

lymphoma Any tumour of the lymphatic tissues.

macrophage A large cell that engulfs and digests cells, micro-organisms and foreign bodies found in the blood stream, connective tissue, bone marrow, lymph, etc.

melanoma A dark-pigmented malignant tumour.

metastasis The aggressively growing, mutated cells that have survived the immune system and migrated, usually by way of the blood stream or the lymphatic system, to set up secondary growth colonies at a distance from the primary tumour in the original cancer mass.

MRI scan Magnetic resonance imaging, using a diagnostic technique that combines radio waves with magnetic forces to produce highly detailed images of the internal structures of the body, both soft tissue and bone structure.

mucilages Gel-like, slimy substances consisting of molecules made up of long chains of sugar units, the complex carbohydrate constituents of many plants. Mucilages have a demulcent and soothing effect when applied to inflamed tissue. The gel is used in some cosmetic preparations.

NK cells Natural killer cells acting as part of the immune system and targeting any cell that displays a tumour antigen. NK cells may be capable of maintaining long-term surveillance of cells in the body, particularly against virus-induced tumours.

oncologist A cancer specialist.

organic As in gardening and foods, grown with fertilizers and mulches consisting only of animal and vegetable matter, with no exposure to chemical fertilizers, herbicides and pesticides.

oxalate Any salt or ester of oxalic acid.

pH values A measure of the acidity or the alkalinity of a solution. 7 = neutral. pH increases with increasing alkalinity (up to 10), decreasing down to zero with increasing acidity.

phenol A basic building block of many plant constituents. Many different phenolic compounds exist that are based upon it.

polysaccharides Sugars that join with other chemicals to produce compounds such as pectin and mucilage which soothe, protect and relax the alimentary canal.

prognosis A forecast of doubtful accuracy based on other people's experiences as to the outcome of an individual disease.

PSA count Prostate-specific antigen, a 'tumour' marker quite specific to the prostate, detected in a blood sample and used to determine malignant cancer levels in the prostate as well as benign cellular changes and prostate inflammation. A rising PSA count does not necessarily mean an automatic cancer diagnosis; initially it may simply indicate that the immune system is active.

purgative glycosides For example, the anthraquinones in Cascara, Senna, Rhubarb and Buckthorn. Salicylic acid often combines with a sugar to form an antiseptic glycoside, as in Meadowsweet.

refrigerant Having cooling or fever-reducing properties.

relaxant Inducing muscle relaxation or relieving tension.

resection The surgical removal of part of an organ or structure.

saponins Glycosides that form a soapy lather when shaken in water. Steroidal saponins appear to mimic the precursors of female sex hormones. Tri-terpenoid saponins appear to mimic the adrenal hormone ACTH.

sarcoma A malignant tumour rising from non-epithelial tissue, such as muscle, blood, fat, etc.

squamous carcinoma Flat, plaque-like cancerous growth derived from the layer of skin cells known as stratified squamous epithelium, typically forming a variable amount of keratin within the tumour (keratin means of hair, nails and horn).

steroid drugs A large group of synthetic drugs; those specific for cancer are generally prescribed to relieve oedema and inflammation.

synergy The action of two or more substances, organs or organisms to achieve a greater effect than the sum of their individual parts.

tannins Compounds that react with protein to produce a leather-like coating on animal tissue similar to the process of tanning. They promote healing and numbing (to reduce irritation), reduce inflammation and halt infection.

T cells T4 cells constitute approximately 55 per cent of the unstimulated T cells in the blood stream; once stimulated they develop into Helper T cells, which are vital in supporting other T cells in the immune system and stimulating B cells into maturation.

T8 cells develop into: (a) Suppressor T cells – as acting to suppress the immune system function, presumably in order to shut down immune system attack on a particular antigen when it ceases to be a threat. Loss of the suppressor function is associated with various auto-immune diseases such as diabetes, lupus and multiple sclerosis;

(b) CTL cells (cytotoxic T lymphocytes) that seem have evolved specifically to attack tumour cells; they are unable to deal with bacteria and parasites and only attack cells with tumour antigens.

virus Any of various submicroscopic pathogens (agents causing disease, as in bacteria or fungus) having the ability to replicate only inside a living cell

vital signs Pulse, breathing, blood pressure and temperature.

volatile oils Complex compounds that are chemical mixtures of hydrocarbons and alcohols. In the living plant, they often enhance the moisture-retaining properties of the leaves. They are the source of the characteristic flavour and taste of many herbs. They have antiseptic, anti-fungal or aromatic properties.

waxes A combination of alcohols and fatty acids.

wild-crafted Herbs that have been harvested from selected places at the correct time of the year.

wild-harvested Herbs harvested from unspecified sites at any time of the year.

Select Bibliography

Badgeley, Laurence, *Healing AIDS Naturally*, Human Energy Press, 1987

Balch, James F. and Phyllis A., *Prescription for Nutritional Healing*, Avery, 1990

Britton, Ted, 'Essiac given most of credit in "miracle birth"', *Examiner*, 1 April 1981

Budwig, Dr Johanna, *Flax Oil as a True Aid Against Arthritis, Heart Infarction, Cancer and other Diseases*, Apple Publishing Co. Ltd, 1994

Cadenas, Enrique and Lester Packer, *Handbook of Antioxidants*, Marcel Dekker, 1996

Caisse, Rene M., R.N. 'I was "Canada's Cancer Nurse"', *The Story of Essiac*, June 1963

The Canadian Journal of Herbalism, vol. 12, no. 3, July 1991

Castleman, Michael, *The Healing Herbs*, Rodale Press, 1991

Christopher, Dr John R., *The School of Natural Healing*, BiWorld, 1976

Clapham, Tutin and Moore, *Flora of the British Isles*, 3rd edn, Cambridge U.P., 1987

The Illustrated Columbia Encyclopedia, Columbia U.P.

The 1975 Corpus Almanac of Canada

Department of Resources and Development, *Native Trees of Canada*, 4th edn, 1950

Dextreit, Raymond, *Our Earth, Our Cure*, Swan House, 1974

D'Mello, J.P. Felix, Carol M. Duffus and John H. Duffus, 'Toxic substances in crop plants', *Royal Society of Chemistry*, 1991

Dorlands Medical Dictionary, 25th edn, W.B. Saunders, 1974

Duke, James A., *Handbook of Medicinal Herbs*, CRC Press, 1986

Epstein, Samuel S. and David Steinman with Susan Le Vert, *The Breast Cancer Prevention Programme*, Macmillan, 1997

Erdmann, Dr Robert and Meirion Jones, *Minerals, The Metabolic Miracle Workers*, 1988

Erichsen-Brown, Charlotte, *Use of Plants for the Past Five Hundred Years*, 1979

Fallon, B. and C.E. Hawtry, 'Pediatric genitourinary neoplasms: clinical, diagnostic and therapeutic features', in *Genitourinary Oncology*, ed. D.A. Culp and S.A. Loening, Lea & Febiger, 1985, pp. 545–70

Fisher, John, *The Origins of Garden Plants*, Constable, 1992

Goldberg, Burton, W. John Diamond M.D. and W. Lee Cowden M.D., *An Alternative Medicine Definitive Guide to Cancer*, Future Medicine, 1997

Grieve, Maude, *A Modern Herbal*, ed. C.F. Leyel, Penguin, 1980

Grimm, W.C., *The Book of Trees*, 1957

Henrikson, Robert, *Earth Food Spirulina*, 1997

Herbal Research Publications, *Naturopathic Handbook of Herbal Formulas*, 1995

Hodgkinson, A., *Oxalic Acid in Biology and Medicine*, Academic Press, 1977

Hoffmann, David, *The Herbal Handbook*, Element, 1987

Hutchens, Alma R., *Indian Herbology of North America*, Shambhala, 1973

Jackson, Mildred and Terri Teague, *The Handbook of Alternatives to Chemical Medicine*, 1975

King, Roger J.B., *Cancer Biology*, 2nd edn, Pearson Education, 2000

Klein, Mali, *A Future Beyond the Sun*, Fisher Miller, 1997

Kloss, Jethro, *Back to Eden*, Woodbridge Press, 1972

Koivister, V.A. and Felig, 'Is skin preparation necessary before insulin injection?', *Lancet*, 1, 1978, 1072–3

Kramer and Koslowski, *Physiology of Woody Plants*, Academic Press, 1979

Kretovich, V.L., *Principles of Plant Biochemistry*, Pergamon Press, 1966

Kruger, Anna, *Herbs*, American Nature Guides, 1992

Kuttan, R. et al., *Cancer Letters*, 29, 1985, 197

Launett, Edwin, *Hamlyn Guide to Edible and Medicinal Plants of Britain and Northern Europe*, Hamlyn, 1981

Lazarides, Linda, *The Waterfall Diet*, Piatkus, 1999

Mills, Simon, *The Dictionary of Modern Herbalism*, Thorsons, 1985

Mills, Simon, *Out of the Earth: The Essential Book of Herbal Medicine*, Viking/Penguin Books, 1991

Mills, Simon, *The Complete Guide to Modern Herbalism*, Thorsons, 1994

Ministry of Natural Resources, Canada, *The Forest Trees of Ontario*, 1986

Moss, Ralph, *Cancer Therapy*, 1992

Mowrey, Daniel B., *The Scientific Validation of Herbal Medicine*, Keats, 1986

National Cancer Institute Journal, Tumour-Damaging Capacity of Plant Material, 1952

Nature Trek Guide, *Wild Herbs of Britain and Europe*

New Age Herbalist, consultant editor Richard Mabey, Gaia Books, 1988

New Internationalist, October 1999, 'The Big Banana Split'; May 2000, 'Pick Your Poison: The Pesticide Scandal'

Olive Enterprises (Muskoka), *The Rene Caisse Story*, VHS colour video, John Newton, 1997

Pedersen, Mark, *Nutrional Herbology*, Pedersen, 1988

Plaskett, Dr Lawrence, *Nutrional Therapy to the Aid of Cancer Patients*, December 1999

Raven, Evert and Eichhorn, *Biology of Plants*, 5th edn, 1992

Reader's Digest, *The Beauty and Splendour of North America*

Reader's Digest, *North American Folk Healing*, 1998

Sams, Jamie, *Sacred Path Cards*, Harper, 1990

Shook, Dr Edward E., *Advanced Treatise on Herbology*, 1934

Snow, Sheila, *The Essence of Essiac*, 1993

Snow, Sheila, *Old Ontario Remedies*, 'Rene Caisse, Essiac', 1991

Snow Fraser, Sheila and Carroll Allen, 'Could Essiac halt cancer?', *Homemakers Magazine*, July 1977

Snow, Sheila and Mali Klein, *The Rene Caisse Formula Interview*, Clouds Trust, 1996

Snow, Sheila and Mali Klein, *Essiac Essentials*, Gill & Macmillan, 1999

Steen, Dr R. Grant, *A Conspiracy of Cells, The Basic Science of Cancer*, Plenum, 1993

Stuart, Malcolm, *The Encyclopaedia of Herbs and Herbalism*, 1987

Thain, M. and M. Hickman, *Penguin Book of Biology*, Penguin, 1996

Tierra, Michael, *Planetary Herbology*, Lotus Press, 1988

Toniolo, P. *et al.*, 'Consumption of meat, animal products, protein and fat, and risk of breast cancer: a prospective cohort study in New York', *Epidemiology*, 5, 4, 1994, 391

USA Today, 'The Great Elm returns', 6 November 1997

US Congress, Office of Technology Assessment (OTA), *Unconventional Cancer Treatments*, Washington, D.C., 1990

Watt, J.M. and Breyer-Brandwijk, *Medicinal and Poisonous Plants of Southern and Eastern Africa*, E&S Livingston, 1962

WDDTY, vol. 10, no. 12, March 2000

Weiner, Michael A. and Janet Weiner, *Herbs that Heal*, 1994

Williams, Kim, *Eating Wild Plants*, Antonson, 1977

Williams, Penny, 'New frontiers', *Homemakers Magazine*, October 1995

World Health Organisation (WHO), *Bull. WHO* (Switzerland), 1989

Youngson, Robert M., *Collins Dictionary of Medicine*, HarperCollins, 1992

Useful Addresses

U.K.

An SAE with all enquiries is appreciated.

For up-to-date information on herbal suppliers:
The Herb Society (Registered Charity No. 265511)
Deddington Hill Farm, Warmington, Banbury, OX17 1XB, UK
Tel. 01295 692000

The National Institute of Medical Herbalists
56, Longbrook Street, Exeter, EX4 6AH, UK
Tel. 01392 426 022

For individual herbs:
The Organic Herb Trading Company (formerly Hambledon Herbs)
Court Farm, Milverton, Somerset TA4 1NF, UK
Tel. 01823 401 205
Fax 01823 401 001
email: info@organicherbtrading.com
http://www.organicherbtrading.com

Information:
Clouds Trust
P.O. Box 30, Liss, Hampshire GU33 7XF, UK
http://www.cloudstrust.org/
Tel. 01730 301162

Essiac on the web: http://www.essiac-info.org/
Rife on the web: http://www.rife.org/

Australia

National Herbalists Association of Australia
49 Oakwood Street, Sutherland, NSW 2232
Tel. 02 92 116 437

Weights and Measures

Liquids

US/CANADA
1 pint = 16 fluid ounces = 0.470 ml
2 US pints = 1 quart = 32 fluid ounces = 0.940 ml
1 American or Canadian cup = 8 fluid ounces = 235 ml
1 gallon = 3.785 litres
1 tablespoon = 0.5 fluid ounce

IMPERIAL/METRIC
60 drops = 1 teaspoon = 5 ml
1 tablespoon = 3 teaspoons = 15 ml = 0.5 fluid ounce
2 tablespoons = 1 fluid ounce
16 tablespoons = 1 cup or 8 fluid ounces
1 pint = 20 fluid ounces = 570 ml
1 gallon = 4.545 litres

Weight

US/CANADA/IMPERIAL/METRIC
1 oz = 28.35 g
16 oz = 1 pound = 455 g = 7,000 grains
US/Canada/UK measurements in pounds and ounces are identical for all practical purposes.

Index